Alkaline Diet

Useful and Simple Guide to Understand PH, apply Herbal Medicine for Fast Weight Loss and Cleanse your body through Exquisite Plant Based Recipes (7 Days Meal Prep)

Marla Wilson

Table Of Contents

Introduction

Staying healthy is not a matter of chance - it is a deliberate choice. It's a choice of what to eat or not eat. We are all faced with this choice on a daily basis, and what we choose is reflected in our overall state of health, because our choices form the internal environment of our body which reflects outwardly.

The notion that germs cause diseases is a flawed premise. We live with and constantly breathe in germs day in and day out. It is not the germs that matter, but the internal environment of our body. It is not mosquitoes that cause ponds to become stagnant, just as maggots, flies, and rats do not cause garbage; they simply feed on garbage. The fact that germs are present in your body does not automatically mean you have a disease. You only get a disease when you create an enabling environment for the germs to thrive.

The question to ask is this: what is your biological terrain like? What you eat and drink creates the terrain – the internal environment – where germs and diseases can either thrive or lie dormant. Have you recently taken a closer look at what you are feeding your body? Are you helping your body maintain health, or are you giving your body excess work through the things you eat and drink?

This book will take you through a

journey that will help you understand the internal workings of your body - how your body constantly struggles under undue pressure caused by poor food choices. You will understand the negative effects of consuming unhealthy foods and drinks; you will also understand why your health deteriorates even though you eat so-called balanced diets.

In this book, I present a balanced perspective of the alkaline diet without unnecessarily exaggerating its capabilities. Misconceptions about what eating an alkaline diet can and cannot do are unbiasedly handled inside this book.

Losing weight seems to top the list of

goals for many people, and they are constantly in search of quicker ways to shed some pounds. Although weight loss is one of the benefits of eating an alkaline diet, this book does not encourage you to use alkaline foods only to lose weight, but to regard the alkaline diet as a key to your overall health. In other words, the ideas presented in this book will encourage you to consider a gradual but complete change in your lifestyle to ensure that whatever benefits you derive from the alkaline diet remain permanent.

The central message of this book is to help your body do its work with ease so as to promote your general well-being. That is why, aside from preaching the alkaline message (devoid of blind sentimentality), I have also included some topics about medicinal herbs that will help you cut down the ingestion of synthetic chemicals and drugs so as not to cause additional damage to your internal environment (biological terrain) in the guise of curing diseases.

Take your time to study this book as you would a guidebook. It is packed with solid common sense that is backed by science and is capable of giving you the health and fitness that you so much desire.

Chapter 1:
Understanding the Basics

A Little Background

I'd like to dive right into showing you the benefits of alkalizing your meals, how to prepare meals that are alkaline friendly, and sharing all the tips and tricks for getting the most out of an alkaline diet - but a little bit of background will be necessary to facilitate our understanding. I am aware that some people reading this book may have some idea about what an alkaline diet is, but for the benefit of those who do not, I'll start by explaining the very basics, which includes what alkaline and pH are.

What is Alkaline?

So, what exactly is alkaline? In simple everyday English, alkaline is a nutrient substance or solution that has a pH above 7 (pH? What is that? Don't worry, we'll get to that soon).

Do you remember acid, base, and salt from back in school? Just in case you don't remember or didn't pay attention back then in class, here's a brief recap.

Acids are substances that contain hydrogen, usually have a sour taste, and form a solution or mixture with a pH value that is below 7. Examples of acids are citric acid (found in lemons and limes), hydrochloric acid (found in apple cider vinegar and black olives), ethanoic or acetic acid (found in canned fruits, mayonnaise, marinades, and other condiments), and sulfuric acid (found in seafood, garlic, onion, peaches, apricots, cheddar, and parmesan cheese).

Bases are substances that neutralize acids. Bases that can dissolve in water or any solvent are known as alkalis or alkaline solutions. A solution can either be acid (acidic) or base (alkaline) depending on its pH. Examples of alkaline are potassium hydroxide (used as food thickeners and food stabilizers), calcium carbonate (found in many ready-to-eat breakfast cereals, almond milk, and cereal bars), and sodium hydroxide or caustic soda (used in ice-creams, chocolates, and pretzels).

When a substance has been neutralized by the reaction between alkali and acid, it forms salt and water.

What is pH?

Ok, I've mentioned pH in more than one place while talking about alkaline. Here's what it means. pH stands for potential of hydrogen. pH level refers to the measure of alkalinity or acidity of a substance, mixture, or solution. The range of pH is measured on a scale from 0 to 14, with 7 being neutral.

That is to say, a pH level of:

- 0.0 to 6.9 is acidic

- 7.0 is neutral (pure water has a pH of 7.0)
- 7.1 – 14.0 is alkaline

Your body tissues and fluids are either acidic or alkaline depending on their pH level. In a normal, healthy person, the overall body is slightly alkaline, with a pH level of between 7.3 and 7.4. However, the pH level of the body varies from organ to organ. Some organs or tissues are more acidic, while others are a bit more alkaline in nature. The most acidic organ in your body is the stomach; this is so because high acid concentration is required to break down the food you eat. The pH level of your blood is somewhere between 7.36 and 7.44; if it falls out of this normal range, it may lead to serious internal damage and possibly sudden death if not corrected quickly.

Maintaining the Body's pH Level

One of the core misconceptions about the alkaline diet centers on the topic of maintaining the body's pH level. The question is: does an alkaline diet maintain the body's pH level, or does the body do all it can to maintain its pH level whether a person is on an alkaline diet or not?

People who do not believe or support the idea of going alkaline insist that the body will always work to keep the pH level balanced. It doesn't require alkaline meals or diets to maintain this balance. After all, it is what the body is naturally designed to do. They view the extra effort of sticking to an alkaline diet as wasted effort and most times, they claim there is not much scientific evidence to back the claim that foods rich in alkaline do actually maintain the body's pH level.

There have also been arguments that the foods we eat ends up in the stomach, which has a high acidity level, and then they are eventually transferred to the intestines where the foods are neutralized by enzymes and digestive liquids. This means the initial pH of whatever food we consume doesn't really matter, because they will all end up having the same pH within our intestines. This is quite a convincing argument, I must say, but is it actually correct? We'll get to that in a bit.

On the other hand, advocates of the alkaline diet swear by the veracity of the diet to help in maintaining the body's pH level. They claim that following an alkaline diet program will ensure that the body's overall pH level stays intact and keep a good number of diseases at bay.

So, where do I stand? Naturally, when you picked up this book, you assumed that I am a diehard fan of anything alkalizing (and you are not far from the truth), but I do like to take my stand based on scientific evidence and not sentiments. So, here's what I know to be the fact.

The idea of eating or following an alkaline diet is not to make the body more alkaline; your body already is. In fact, your blood is always alkaline and your intelligent body will do all it can to keep it that way. In that respect, antagonists of the alkaline diet are correct.

On the flip side, your body does work – serious work, to keep itself in the normal alkaline state. There is constant filtering, detoxifying, and neutralizing going on that in the long-run may cause too much stress for your body and eventually reduce its efficiency in maintaining your overall good health and well-being. However, you can ease this workload by eating foods that are not too acidic. That is to say, eating an alkaline diet will ensure that the body does its work of maintaining the pH level without much stress. Hence, the effort required by the body is minimal, which means your body energy and resources are conserved for other important things. In this regard, advocates of the alkaline diet are correct when they say alkaline foods help the body to maintain its pH level.

If you understand this balanced view, you will no longer be caught in between the crossfire of arguments for or against the alkaline diet. This is one of the benefits of studying this book – I present to you a balanced and unbiased perspective about alkaline diet not just from my point of view, but from a scientific and logical standpoint. However, because I do not wish to make this book into an academic material, I will cut down on the presentation of research (since, for many people, scientific studies are very boring to read!).

Later, we shall take a look at what foods are required to help the body in its work of maintaining the body's pH level. For now, let us give our attention to how you can test your body's pH level. And yes, it is something you can do at home without necessarily going for a laboratory test.

But before we discuss how to test our pH, let's go back to the view that says the initial pH of the foods we eat doesn't matter because they all end up with the same pH as our intestinal fluids; the question is, how comes the pH levels of our external fluids (urine and saliva) vary with the foods we eat? The result of all pH tests for urine and saliva should remain the same if the foods we eat have no effect on our overall pH level, don't you think? The mere fact that the types of food we eat show up in our pH test results should tell you that your food does, in fact, affect your overall pH level to some extent. If you take the time to deliberately choose what types of food to eat for just a few weeks and then monitor your pH through regular testing, you will come to the same conclusion as many others have - that the initial pH of your food is very important to your overall health.

I may not agree with every single "miraculous" claim about eating alkaline foods, but this much is true: what you eat matters a lot, and it affects your health in more ways than you may realize.

Testing Your Body's pH Level

Whether it is out of curiosity or necessity, I recommend that before you begin an alkaline diet, you should test your pH level. There is a possibility of over-alkalinity in the body, and that is a state you really don't want to be in. Later, we shall discuss the possibility of excess alkalinity in the body. So, to avoid hurting yourself in a bid to stay healthy, I strongly advise that you take the simple test.

But earlier on, I did mention that your blood pH level rarely changes and if does, it is very likely to result in death. Since this is so, what is the point in testing the body's pH level? If you are alive (you have to be if you are reading this book!), your blood's pH is fine and testing it will make no difference. Or will it?

Well, to be clear, testing your body's pH level by itself doesn't change anything, but it does tell you something useful: continue your eating habits or change your eating habits. Furthermore, the purpose of testing your pH level is not to know your blood pH level. It is to know the pH level of your body's external fluids, organs, and cells. Earlier, I did mention that your body's pH differs from organ to organ. That is because the blood keeps itself constantly at the same pH level and dumps all the other acidity into the organs, cells, and other external fluids of your body. In other words, to keep you alive, the blood constantly purges toxins (acidity) out of itself and deposits them into other parts of your body. If you do not test to know the pH level of these other parts of your body, you may have a health disaster waiting to happen.

In summary, the message I am trying to convey is that your body is exposed to diseases if you neglect to maintain the pH balance of your body's external fluids, cells, and organs. And you certainly cannot know this without testing your body's (not blood's) pH level.

There are several inexpensive ways to test your pH level. The common ones are the saliva test and the urine test. For both tests, you will need to purchase a box of pH test strips or indicator strips from a drugstore (for a more accurate reading, use the pH test strips instead of pH test paper). The strips are scientifically calibrated to show you the pH level. The test strips usually have colored keys or charts printed on the back of each strip or on the back of the box so that you can easily interpret your test result.

The Saliva Test

The pH level of your saliva is closely related to the pH of the fluids around your cells (known as interstitial fluids). This means that the saliva test is likely to show you how good or poor your diet is and what your body's general pH is. When your body is generally low on alkaline levels, your blood starts to "steal" from your bones, joints, and bodily fluids like the saliva. In that case, your alkaline levels will come up low on a saliva test, which is a clear warning for you to either eat less acidic foods and drinks or consume more alkaline foods and drinks.

Follow these simple steps to take the saliva test:

1. Wiggle your tongue inside your mouth to stimulate saliva.

2. When there is sufficient saliva in your mouth, spit it out or swallow.

3. Fill up your mouth with saliva again and spit it onto a plastic spoon or directly on the test strip.

4. Allow the strip to remain in your

spit for about 3 seconds if you dipped the strip into a spoon containing your spit before taking it out.

5. Wait for about 15 seconds to see the color of the strip.

6. Use the chart on the back of the strip or strip box to interpret the result of your test.

Optimal Saliva Test Result

The optimal saliva pH is 7.2 or slightly higher, however, saliva pH can rise to 7.8 after eating. Here are some simple guidelines to help you determine what your saliva test result means. These are:

• Healthy children will have a reading of between 7.0 and 7.5 pH

- Healthy adults should have a reading of anywhere between 6.8 and 7.2 pH

- Although there may not be any apparent illness, a consistent level of 6.8 pH in an adult shows a strong indication of alkaline deficiency.

- An adult with a reading of 6.5 pH is deficient.

- A reading of 4.5 pH indicates a severe deficiency and the adult is most likely to have a serious disease (like cancer).

The Urine Test

The pH level of your urine indicates how well your kidneys, gonads, lungs, and adrenals are performing to keep too much acidity out of your body through buffers (minerals) and hormones.

To perform the urine test is actually simple. Just follow the steps below:

1. Begin with your first morning urine before you eat or drink anything.

2. Simply urinate in your usual way and wait for a steady stream to start. Then wet the strip in the stream of urine for about 2 to 3 seconds.

3. Shake off excess urine from the strip (gently of course, you don't want to splash urine everywhere!) and wait for about 15 seconds.

4. Use the chart on the back of the

strip or strip box to interpret the result of your test.

Optimal Urine Test Result

Optimally, urine pH should range from 6.5 to about 7.2 in a normal healthy person. It may be lower in the mornings but tends to go higher later in the day or towards the evenings. This is because urine pH is affected by factors such as:

- The types of foods and drinks you consume
- The preservatives in the foods you eat
- The quantity of water you drink
- Pollutants you inhale
- The quality of sleep and rest you get

- The amount of stress you encounter

- The pathogens present in your body

- And the various biochemical activities taking place inside your body

However, digestive enzymes do not affect urine pH, as they affect saliva pH.

Recommendations

1. Performing a pH test shouldn't be a one-off thing. For you to reach any meaningful conclusion, I strongly recommend that you perform the urine or saliva test for a 30-day period. This will show you a clear trend or pattern so that you

know exactly what your body is telling you. A one-time test shows you just a pixel in the entire picture; a continuous test over a long period shows you the entire picture!

2. Please do not put the test strip directly into your mouth when doing the saliva test. This is not ideal. I've seen a lady put the test strip directly into her mouth, and to make matters worse, she closed her lips when pulling out the test strip. Does the sex of person have anything to do with the saliva test? Actually, no. But women tend to have lipstick on. So closing your lips while pulling out the test strip when you have lipstick on will likely smear

on the test strip and mess with your result. But aside from smearing lipstick on the test strips, you are not supposed to ingest the substances (chemicals) on the test strip. So spit on the test strip or on a plastic spoon and dip the test strip into it for best results.

3. The saliva test should be done at least 2 hours after eating your last meal or drinking anything. Testing your pH using the saliva method right after eating will give you a very wrong result. You are simply going to get the result of what you just ate or drank.

4. Do not brush your teeth before taking the saliva test.

5. Your first urine after you wake up contains the deposits of metabolic acids which were stored in your bladder throughout the night. Therefore, it is normal for the test result of your first urine of the day to be slightly acidic. Usually, your second urine of the day (before you eat any food) would show you your ideal urine pH level.

What Do You Do If Your Saliva or Urine pH is Below Optimum Levels?

This book is basically designed to help you shift from an acidic pH level to a slightly alkaline pH level. That's my way of saying that if your pH level is below optimum, you should implement the ideas in this book. However, here are some quick tips you can use to effect some changes in your pH level if your saliva and urine tests don't measure up to the optimal alkaline levels.

1. Drink Alkaline Water

Drinking alkaline water will help to improve your body's alkaline buffering capability. It is a great way to flush out acidic wastes from your body. Drinking alkaline water is also a good way to keep the body hydrated.

2. Increase Your Intake of Alkaline Foods

Basically, if you are deficient in alkaline, the general rule is to ensure that your daily meals are made up of about 80% alkaline foods and only 20% acidic foods. That means you should cut down on foods like fish and meat, and significantly reduce the rate you consume sugary soft drinks, because these are all classified as strongly acidic foods. Nuts, legumes, and grains are mildly acidic; be cautious of how you consume them. Your focus should be on foods that are mildly alkaline like berries, vegetables, and fruits. Equally, spinach, broccoli, and green leafy vegetables can be consumed in moderate amounts too, as they are considered strongly alkaline. In a later chapter, we shall take a look at a comprehensive list of acidic and alkaline foods.

3. Include Freshly Made Juices in Your Meals

You simply cannot get enough nutrients from your meals to beat the number of nutrients you drink from freshly made juices packed full of healthy vegetables and fruits. Form the habit of drinking freshly homemade juices to provide adequate mineral buffers for your body.

4. Increase Your Intake of Alkaline Minerals

Consider increasing your consumption of alkaline salts like potassium bicarbonate, rubidium, and cesium. The next time you want to bake, opt for potassium bicarbonate instead of sodium bicarbonate (commonly called baking soda). You can also add a teaspoon of potassium bicarbonate into your water and drink it every night just before retiring for the day.

5. Do Not Brush Your Teeth Too Soon

When you consume foods or drinks that are high in acidic content, avoid brushing your teeth soon afterward. Beverages like beer, wine, and cider have high acidity levels and can make your tooth enamel soft. This is why brushing too soon after consuming any of these can be damaging to your enamel. Black coffee is also highly acidic, but you can add some dairy to it to reduce the acidity; just make sure it is not a creamer that is sugary.

6. Chew A Sugarless Gum

Chewing gum that contains xylitol will stop bacteria from getting stuck to your enamel. Besides, chewing gum can improve your pH balance by boosting saliva production.

Bottom Line

Keeping close tabs on your pH level (through testing) will give you early signs of imbalance in your system. Your intelligent body gives you messages on a daily basis; take advantage of these messages so that you can take steps to either improve or maintain your pH balance.

In Summary...

We've covered quite some grounds in this opening chapter. Below is a quick recap of the major points:

- Alkaline is a substance with a pH above 7.
- pH measures the acidity or alkalinity of a substance. A reading below 7 is acidic, above 7 is alkaline, and a reading of 7 is neutral. Pure water has a pH of 7.
- Our body has a pH level ranging between 7.3 and 7.4. Different

organs and body fluids have varying pH levels, but our blood has a constant range of pH. The slightest deviation from that level may signal death.

- The body works tirelessly to make sure it maintains a steady pH. The more acidic things we ingest, the more work it does.

- We can help take off some workload by reducing the acidic foods we eat.

- Saliva and urine can reveal the pH of our internal organs and fluids. Using test strips can reveal whether we have balanced pH levels or not.

Chapter 2: The Alkaline Diet

Alkaline Diet: What Is It?

We've spent an entire chapter trying to lay the foundation for the subject of the alkaline diet. It is a nice background to have so that we'll not be going back and forth in a bid to explain what the alkaline diet is all about. And now that we have the foundation out of the way, let's see what the alkaline diet actually is.

So, what exactly is the alkaline diet?

The way I see the alkaline diet is slightly different from a typical alkaline fan. Here's how I define the alkaline diet: *an alkaline diet is a set of meals designed to help in* **reducing the amount of work done by your body** *to balance its pH level by reducing the intake of acidic foods while increasing the consumption of alkalizing foods.*

But what is the difference between this definition and the typical alkaline diet definition? Well, there's not much difference except that my emphasis is on helping the body with its work of balancing the body's pH. Some other definitions tend to imply that the body's pH will not be balanced without eating an alkaline diet; that is not entirely correct. The body will do all it can to maintain its pH, especially in the blood, even if it means doing extra hard work.

What an alkaline diet does is to reduce the consumption of high acid-forming foods which will require neutralizing when they get into our bodies.

Basically, following an alkaline diet would mean going through your food and drink list and striking out those that are high in acid. The problem is that many of the foods and drinks we like to consume have very high acidity levels. Accumulating too much acidity in your body will strain the body in its normal functioning, sapping you of energy and lowering your body's immune function. We all are aware that low immunity means a higher chance of letting diseases take over.

In the previous chapter, we said alkaline substances are those with pH above 7. So, foods that have pH below 7 are acidic, and consuming too much of them over a long period of time may make you vulnerable to all kinds of diseases.

But do acidic foods really hurt the body? Should we completely eliminate acids from our food and body? Well, first of all, it is impossible to completely eliminate acids from your body, even if you may succeed in doing so with foods which, by the way, is not in your best interest! Your stomach, for example, is full of a high concentration of acids, and that is a very good thing because, without acids, your stomach would not be able to break down your foods.

Acids do not hurt our bodies, a fact that many alkaline diet proponents seem to ignore. The focus of the alkaline diet is to balance your acidity and alkalinity levels; it is not to eliminate one in favor of the other! Too much acidity is not healthy for your body - neither is too much alkalinity. It is very crucial to understand this point, because it is central to the whole concept of eating an alkaline diet.

Having said that, it is important to point out that the emphasis on decreasing acidic food consumption is present because we eat too much of them to the exclusion of alkaline forming foods. Hence, there is imbalance or lopsidedness in our eating habit. But just in case you have doubts about reducing your intake of acid-forming foods, here's a quick summary of what too much acidity can do to your body over a long period.

Side Effects of Prolonged Excess Acidity

- Aching muscles and joint pain
- A buildup of lactic acid
- Bladder conditions and the possibility of developing kidney stones
- Chronic inflammation
- High blood pressure
- Chronic fatigue and low energy

- Mood swings
- Slow metabolism
- Inability to shed weight leading to obesity
- Diabetes and weight gain
- Weak bones, osteoporosis, bone spurs, and fractures
- Premature aging
- Slow digestion and elimination
- Weakened immunity
- Yeast/fungal overgrowth

These health conditions are enough motivation to propel anyone towards reducing their intake of highly acidic foods and drinks. The main reason why most people suffer from these conditions is poor diet. Other reasons include inadequate exercise, too many stress-inducing workouts (like excess cardio), and chronic stress. All of these are capable of causing our internal environment to become highly acidic. When this happens, minerals like calcium, sodium, potassium, and magnesium will begin to "migrate" from our bones and other vital organs of the body to help in neutralizing the excess acid to keep the body's pH balance. This is an anomaly in the body's metabolic process, and if left unattended for a long time, it can lead to any or more of the above health conditions.

Before I discuss how to get into the process of alkalizing your diet properly, let's take a quick detour to see how metabolic wastes affect the acidity and alkalinity of our body.

Metabolic Wastes

The process of breaking down food into energy – metabolism – is much like burning something in a fire. When something is burnt, it leaves ash residues behind. Equally, when food is converted into energy through metabolism, wastes or "metabolic ash" is left behind.

But wait, I am not just making this up. Back in the 1870s, the Bomb Calorimeter was used by Marcellin Berthelot, a scientist, to burn different types of foods. He found that by mixing the ash of the burnt food with water, he could determine the pH of the food[1]. He observed that most vegetables, fruits, and many plant-based items were more alkaline, while processed foods and meats were more acidic. Berthelot's work actually laid the foundation for the alkaline diet.

It is not surprising, therefore, to hear people refer to the alkaline diet as "*the alkaline ash diet*". The metabolic process that converts your foods to energy always deposits an acidic ash residue or alkaline ash residue in your body as metabolic waste. And since most of us are always eating almost on a daily basis, you can imagine the amount of "ash" your metabolic system leaves

---

[1] Encyclopedia.com (2008). Berthelot, Pierre Eugène Marcellin https://www.encyclopedia.com/people/science-and-technology/chemistry-biographies/pierre-eugene-marcellin-berthelot

behind in your body on a daily basis. If the foods you eat leave behind acidic ash, it simply means your body has more acidity; the opposite is true if you eat foods that leave behind alkaline ash. In other words, the foods you eat can either alkalize your body or acidify your body. Please note that I am referring to your overall body pH and not your blood. The foods you eat do not change your blood's pH.

Alkaline ash in the body is okay and helps to even keep diseases away. On the other hand, too much acid ash in the body leaves you vulnerable to diseases and illnesses. With the types of foods and drinks readily available in most of our modern societies, it is now "normal" for us to eat foods that deposit acidic ash in our bodies. It's little wonder a lot of people are becoming obese and finding it difficult to maintain their health and fitness. To make matters worse, the multi-million dollar fast food businesses are constantly in our faces, enticing us with yummy commercials. Thankfully, we can deliberately take back the control of our health and fitness through the types of foods we choose to consume and the amount of body movement we incorporate into our daily activities.

Alkalizing Your Diet: The Process

First things first: take it slow! It is normal to be excited about starting a new diet plan, and with this excitement comes high expectations, too. But before you rush into taking every acid-forming food out of your meals, remember that for change to be sustainable, it has to be a gradual process. Begin by taking baby steps; incremental changes are better than being dramatic about your diet change, which usually doesn't last. You are more likely to stick to the alkaline diet if you change gradually.

Here are steps I strongly recommend you follow to alkalize your diet. Keep in mind to always test your pH on a regular basis while you are changing your diet.

Step 1: Eat Whole Foods

The foundation for alkalizing your food is to focus on eating plant-based foods.

It is even more preferable if you can get whole foods grown organically. This means you are going to gradually shift from eating all the junk (fast foods) and sugary foods you are used to, and focus on foods like fresh fruits and vegetable, vegetable juices, fermented foods, sprouts of grains, freshly squeezed fruit juices, vegetables (lightly steamed), and toasted nuts, among others. These types of foods are very good at helping your digestion, as they retain active enzymes. Try as much as possible to eat foods (especially vegetables and fruits) in their raw form. When you cook foods, you reduce their alkalizing minerals.

But do not limit yourself to eating the same types of foods over and over again. It is a good practice to expand your food choices, as this will give you nutritional variety. The final chapter of this book contains quite a number of foods you can experiment with, although it is not an exhaustive list.

Step 2: Increase Your Intake of Alkaline-Forming Foods by 60 – 80%

The next thing to do is to concentrate on eating alkaline-forming foods. If your health is dwindling or your immune system is having some sort of problem, I suggest you increase your alkaline food consumption to about 80%. That means only 20% of your daily foods should be mildly acidic or neutral. But if you are looking to maintain already good health, I'd recommend that you keep your intake of alkaline-forming foods to about 60%. So, from now on, when you are shopping for food, create your shopping list from the chart you'll find in the final chapter of this book.

Step 3: Eat Foods that are Good for Your Immune System

Eating foods that your immune system reacts to negatively is not healthy for you. It is important to identify foods that are unsuitable for your immune system (even if they are healthy foods).

Step 4: Follow A Healthy Ratio of Eating Macronutrients

Carbohydrates, fats, and proteins are the major macronutrients in the foods you eat. Maintaining a healthy ratio of these macronutrients in your meal is vital for alkalizing your diet. Use the following to guide you:

Carbohydrates (whole foods): Let your daily meals consist of 60 to 70% plant-based carbohydrates like whole grains, vegetables, and legumes (lentils, peas, and beans). Herbs, spices, and seasonings also fall into this category.

Fats: Consider eating about 15 to 20% of healthy fats per day. By healthy fats, I am referring to omega-3 essential fats that can help your body in the production of energy, protein, and the repair of body tissues. Excellent food sources of healthy fats are foods like olive oil, walnuts, avocados, deep-sea fish oils, sesame, safflower, and peanuts. However, because it may not be possible to make adequate amounts of healthy fats available in your meals (eating deep-sea fish oils at least thrice every week), I will recommend that you take unadulterated omega-3 supplements.

Keep in mind, however, that hydrogenated oils and trans fats are not good for your body, so avoid them. It is difficult to avoid trans fat in these days of too many processed foods, French fries, and the likes unless you are willing to go the extra mile to avoid fast foods. Ensure you use unsaturated and organic oils for cooking your meals. Solid cooking fats like lard, hydrogenated vegetable oil, and margarine are off limits because they are artificial and negatively impact immune function. They have also been linked with high levels of cholesterol since they are capable of interfering with the enzymes in your liver.

Protein: 15 – 20% protein is considered adequate for daily consumption. You can get quality protein from dairy products, eggs, whey protein, and fishes like salmon, tuna, sardines, herring, and mackerel. You can also get protein from foods like mushrooms, miso, seeds and nuts, nutritional yeasts, and sprouts.

Additionally, you can pair foods to get quality protein. This is a good way to create "complete protein" since plant proteins tend to be deficient in some vital amino acids. This means some plants, when eaten alone, do not provide adequate protein, for example, brown rice. But when combined with another plant protein like beans (which also is incomplete protein by itself), it will provide a complete protein as both foods will complement each other. So, it is a good practice to combine or pair foods like:

- Rice and beans

- Corn, rice, and beans

- Legumes and seeds

- Dairy with nuts

- Dairy with grains

- Grains with legumes, seeds, dairy, or nuts

Step 5: Eat Lots of Fiber and Drink Adequate Amounts of Water

Aim to keep your daily fiber intake to about 40 grams at the least. Fibers are roughages that help to shorten the time it takes for foods we eat to transit from stomach to waste elimination. They also make waste elimination easy, thereby keeping your system free of toxic waste elements.

Water is very vital to the proper functioning of your body. There is hardly any part or system in your body that does not depend on water in order to function optimally. To begin with, you shouldn't eat plenty of fiber without matching it with corresponding plentiful water. Consuming adequate water will ensure that the fiber you eat moves wastes efficiently through your body.

Aim for at least 8-ounce of pure water about 8 times per day. You can add fresh lime or lemon juice to your drinking water. They not only enhance the taste of your water, they equally serve as alkaline enhancers and aid digestion. I'd also recommend that, to allow proper digestion, you do not drink water 30 minutes or thereabout before and after you eat your meals. But if it is necessary to drink water when you eat or within the 30 minutes before and after eating, do make sure you drink a very small amount. Also, it should not be cold water – room temperature is ideal. Hot water or tea (healthy tea) can also be consumed. Your digestion can be slowed down if you drink cold water. What about the popular alkaline water: should you drink it or not? Does it work, or is it just market hype? In the next chapter, I shall briefly discuss alkaline water. For starters, simply ensure that you drink enough water throughout your day.

Step 6: Watch Your Food Combinations

Improper food combinations can have a serious negative impact on your overall health. For your nutrition to be considered balanced, you need to ensure that your food combinations are suitable for your digestion and also minimize any adverse effect on your digestive system. If you are vulnerable to having a leaky gut, acid reflux, heartburn, bloating, irritable bowel, or any other digestive discomforts, you need to pay particular attention to the types of foods you combine regardless of whether they are healthy foods or not.

Step 7: Consume Energy Drinks that are Natural

A lot of the so-called energy-boost drinks available are heavily laden with sugar and caffeine, which end up creating more acidic contents in your body. Opt for natural energy giving drinks like lemon water, peppermint tea, or you can take any green powder supplement that is capable of buffering excess acids in your system, stimulate your metabolism, and as well cleanse your digestive system.

Step 8: Cut Down Consumption of Alcohol

I know this may be a tricky one for many people, but I am not suggesting that you completely give up alcohol (although that's not such a bad idea!). You see, the truth is that most alcoholic drinks contain high amounts of sugar. This makes them very acidic and not very suitable for your body, especially when consumed in excess or frequently. Drinking alcohol "once in a blue moon" won't hurt you, however, these things have a way of becoming a habit. So, keep your guard up!

But just in case you do not know what risk you are putting your body through when you consume alcohol, take a look at the list below:

- **Inability to quickly burn fat**: alcohol messes with the functions of your liver – one of the major organs that help you burn fat (in order to lose weight), expel hormonal wastes, and aid in detoxification. If you are really committed to your goal of losing weight, you will have to bid a temporary farewell to alcohol.

- **Depletion of vitamins**: regular intake of alcohol can lead to a fast depletion in your vitamins, especially vitamin B since it is required to break down the alcohol. When vitamin B is lacking in your body, you will experience intense hangovers, increased anxiety levels, and you become vulnerable to general stress.

- **Lack of quality sleep**: you may be thinking that alcohol will make you sleep well, right? Wrong! True, you may get drowsy faster with alcohol, but getting a deep, restful night's sleep will always elude you because the effect of alcohol-induced sleep is very short-lived. Sleep interruption often occurs when you drink alcohol because your body metabolizes alcohol during your sleep time. One ounce of alcohol may take roughly an hour to metabolize, therefore, drinking alcohol especially towards bedtime may disrupt your sleep, and a frequent occurrence can lead to sleep disorders.

- **Affects your skin**: over a long time, alcohol consumption may lead to the dilation of your facial blood vessels, which will eventually result in having spider-like veins showing up on your face, especially around your nose. Also, too much alcohol can cause excess oil to be stimulated due to an imbalance between testosterone and estrogen levels in your body. This can result in pimples. Wrinkles can also result from the dehydration arising from too many glasses of wine. In short, too much alcohol is not a good fit for your skin. Water is a far better option to keep your skin youthful and to maintain an even complexion.

Bottom line: If you are really determined to get the best out of alkalizing your diet, take the extra step of cutting alcohol consumption down to a minimum.

Step 9: Exercise

Sweat has a pH range between 4.5 and 7.0 in a normal, healthy person. This means when we sweat, we allow acid out of our bodies. Although this has nothing to do with eating an alkaline diet, it still has something to do with creating an acid-alkaline balance in the body. So, go ahead and include exercise as part of your lifestyle. Working out for at least 20 to 30 minutes for a minimum of 3 times a week is a great way to live. Moreover, if you are seeking to shed some weight, it is vital to shift from a sedentary lifestyle to a more deliberately active lifestyle. In a later chapter, we shall take a look at how the alkaline diet can help you lose weight... fast!

There you have it! Follow the steps above and you will have alkalized your diet. Remember, the key to sustainable results is consistency. You cannot be consistent if you begin with giant strides. Begin small and take it a step at a time. Your body is used to eating certain types of foods for a very long time; it only makes sense to introduce change in a gradual manner.

One of the reasons why people jump from one diet program to another is lack of patience. No diet can give you the result you seek overnight. Give the alkaline diet a shot for about 30 days, remembering to regularly test your pH levels, and you will be amazed at the results you get within that time if you remain consistent and follow the recommended food types. To help you out, I have included a 7-Day Meal Prep in Chapter 7 of this book to guide you on what to eat for the very first week. Feel free to be creative and choose from the list of foods from the food chart in Chapter 8 to prepare your meals. Losing weight may be your primary goal for getting into an alkaline diet program, however, you will quickly discover that the health benefits of eating an alkaline diet go far beyond just weight loss. And on that note, let us take a moment to consider the various benefits of eating an alkaline diet in the next chapter.

In Summary...

As we are getting ready to see the health benefits of this amazing diet, let's have a quick review of what we have learned so far in this chapter.

- The alkaline diet is a way of eating that helps to ease the work neutralizing acids by the body
- We do not aim to completely eliminate acids from our meals but to find a balance between the

acidity and alkalinity of our bodies.

- Most of the foods we are used to eating are highly acidic and cause harm to our bodies.

- When our foods are broken down, the metabolic wastes or ash that is produced affects our body pH. Eating foods that are high in acids creates a deposit of acidic ash in our bodies, which is not really healthy for our system.

- Significantly cutting down the intake of these foods and increasing our consumption of alkaline-forming foods will shift the overall balance of your body's pH to its natural equilibrium.

- Accumulation of excess acids in

the body for long periods of time can cause weight gain, diabetes, chronic inflammation, premature aging, fungal overgrowth, and slow metabolism among many other health conditions.

- Eating whole foods, taking into cognizance the proper ratio of macronutrients, and consuming adequate amounts of fiber and water are among the steps required to alkalize your diet.

- If you cannot completely avoid alcohol, then by all means, reduce your intake by a significant measure.

Chapter 3: Health Benefits of The Alkaline Diet

What makes the alkaline diet stand out from other diets? Losing weight? If losing weight is the only benefit of eating an alkaline diet, you may as well follow any other diet program out there – and there are quite a number of them that promise weight loss. However, weight loss is but one of the several benefits that are derivable from following the alkaline diet, and I've written this chapter to show you how alkalizing your meals can improve your overall health. As I mentioned in the introduction of this book, staying healthy is not so much a matter of not having germs in our bodies as it is making the internal and external environment of our bodies unsuitable for germs to breed. As you will find with the benefits listed below, highly acidic environments are breeding grounds for pathogens.

The Alkaline Diet: Benefits

1. **Significantly reduces inflammation and chronic pain**: chronic pains like joint pain, back pain, muscle spasms, menstrual symptoms, and chronic inflammation are all linked to acidosis (excess acidity in the body). Restoring the acid-alkaline balance of the body by following an alkaline diet can help to

greatly alleviate chronic inflammation and pains.

2. **Improves digestion**: indigestion, gastric reflux, bloating, nausea, and other digestive disorders are prompted by low alkaline minerals inside our intestinal tracts. This simply means that our gastric region has excess acid. Eating alkaline-forming foods produces alkaline minerals that help the pancreas so it can correctly signal the body about what to do with the foods we eat. In the absence of alkaline minerals, the pancreas can get exhausted and fail to pass the appropriate message to the body. This can result in organs becoming inflamed as well as digestive

problems.

3. **Helps to maintain a healthy weight**: by significantly reducing inflammation and leptin levels, alkaline-forming foods will keep your body from gaining weight by improving the fat-burning process. We shall discuss more on weight loss in a subsequent chapter.

4. **Improves the urinary system**: our kidneys are the main organs in the urinary system. Their main task is to filter fluids and to keep the blood purified. Excess acidity in the body can cause alkaline minerals to be taken from other parts of the body to the blood. Here's the thing: a frequent occurrence of this movement

of alkaline minerals from other parts to your blood means that there is extra purifying and filtering to be done by your kidneys. Eventually, there would be a buildup of alkaline minerals in your kidneys, and that would lead to kidney stones. Adequate consumption of alkaline-forming foods gives the kidneys less work to do and guards against kidney stones.

5. **Prevents stroke and hypertension**: an alkaline diet promotes the production of growth hormones. This function offers protection against hypertension, strokes, memory loss, and high cholesterol. As a matter of fact, an alkaline diet has anti-aging effects on

the body.

6. **Promotes a healthy and even skin tone**: rashes and pimples on the skin can result from an imbalance of the body's pH. The acid buildup causes inflammation, which makes the skin vulnerable to infections. This is what leads to skin eruptions (pimples).

7. **Helps the circulatory system**: excess internal acidity can lead to heart disease. This happens when arteries begin to thicken with fatty plaques in response to inflammation caused by an excess internal acidic environment. This thickening of the arteries happens so as to prevent leaks that can lead to

death, however, the downside is that it puts a lot of strain on the heart, as it narrows the path through which blood flows. When this strain becomes too much for the heart to bear and the heart becomes too exhausted, a situation called a heart attack occurs. This can be averted by keeping internal acidity low, as it naturally should be.

8. **Boosts muscle performance**: have you ever seen someone breathing heavily just by performing some sort of simple tasks, for example, walking and talking at the same time? That's probably because there is an inefficient delivery of oxygen to their body cells - a clear

symptom of abnormally high acidity (acidosis). Too much acidity in the cells of your muscles can interrupt the breakdown of oxygen and glucose into energy. In other words, an acidic environment is not ideal for optimal performance of your muscles. On the flip side, an alkaline environment leads to adequate aerobic metabolism and energy supply to the body.

9. **Guards against respiratory problems**: just as you breathe, your cells too breathe. But they cannot breathe properly when the movement of oxygen is strangulated by excess acidity in body tissues and organs. When there is an imbalance in the ratio of acid-alkaline in our respiratory

organs in favor of acids, it causes wastes like viruses, infections, and mucus to build up in our lungs. This can result in asthma, bronchitis, and colds.

10. **Prevents magnesium deficiency and increases vitamin absorption**: an alkaline diet provides your body with adequate amounts of alkaline minerals like potassium, calcium, and magnesium. These are essential for several functions of the body. Magnesium particularly is required for the smooth functioning of hundreds of bodily processes and enzyme systems. A deficiency in

magnesium can result in frequent headaches, muscle pains, heart complications, anxiety, and sleep disorders. Magnesium also helps the body to easily absorb vitamins like vitamin D, which is central to proper endocrine and immune functioning.

11. **Promotes healthy and strong bones**: a significant increase in bone mineral density can be directly traced to a decrease in acid load which comes with eating alkaline-forming foods. This means you develop healthy and strong bones by following an alkaline diet plan. Have you ever wondered what the word arthritis means? In case you do not know, it simply means inflammation of the

joint. The most common forms of arthritis (which, by the way, is a common disease even in developed countries) are osteoarthritis and rheumatoid. And guess what? They are both linked to the accumulation of acids in the joints and pH imbalance. When acids are accumulated in the joints, it causes damage to the cartilage because the fluids which are supposed to lubricate the joints are now acidic, and this leads to irritation that swells up the joints. To protect your bone density, it is advisable to consume adequate amounts of alkaline-forming vegetables and fruits; this will ensure proper bone structure maintenance.

12. **Improves the nervous system**: your emotional, mental, and physical body requires energy to function properly. Excess acidity in the body deprives it of this vital energy and causes enervation – a situation where your body becomes excessively weak. Alkaline minerals restore proper energy circulation in the body, thus injecting life and vitality to the body.

13. **Boosts immune system**: if the environment is not conducive for a germ, it dies. Conversely, if the germ finds a good breeding ground, it thrives. Disease-causing agents (pathogens) thrive in acidic environments. Therefore, if you consistently laden your body with

excess acid-forming foods (like most people in the western world do), you are simply creating a breeding ground for germs! I do not mean to suggest that pathogens or bad bacteria cannot live in your body if you eat alkaline-forming foods; what I am emphasizing is the fact that pathogens cannot thrive in such a body. You do not fall sick because of the presence of bad bacteria in your body; falling sick is a result of an imbalance in your internal system.

Common Foods that "Influence" Body pH Level

I have said before that what you eat cannot change your pH (especially your blood pH), but it can help your body maintain your pH level by reducing the need to overexert itself in the process of neutralizing too much acidity. In this section, I'll show you a few of the common foods that can influence the body's pH either positively (alkalizing) or negatively (acidifying). And I am using the word "influence" here with caution, because I wouldn't want you to misconstrue that to mean change your body's pH level.

Alkaline Foods You Need to Eat More of

There are some groups of foods that are considered top alkaline foods which you definitely have to include in your diet if you really want to alkalize your meals. Increasing the consumption of these foods will ensure that you enjoy the health benefits we have outlined above. These groups of foods are:

- **Fresh vegetables and fruits**: topping the list of fresh vegetable and fruits are avocado, spinach, broccoli, cucumber, barley grass, wheat grass, alfalfa grass, cabbage, green beans, jicama, kale, figs, mushroom, oregano, ginger, garlic, ripe banana, watermelon, summer black radish, tomatoes, raisins, dates, citrus, grapefruit, red beet, celery, and endive.
- **Plant-based proteins**: eat proteins from plants like almonds,

lima beans, and navy beans. Also, tempeh, tofu, and edamame, which are fermented soy products, are good sources of plant-based proteins.

- **Green drinks**: juices made from freshly squeezed green vegetables or from ground grasses are full of chlorophyll and are alkaline-forming foods.

- **Anti-inflammatory herbs and spices**: consider using the following spices and herbs for your meals: turmeric, ginger, cloves, cinnamon, cayenne, rosemary, sage, spirulina, and black pepper

- **Most seeds and nuts**: these include cardamom seeds, cumin seeds, fennel seeds, flaxseed, and pumpkin seeds. There are some excellent seeds and nuts, too, which may not be categorized as alkaline foods but which are neither acidic either. These neutral seeds and nuts include cashews, chestnuts, hazelnuts, macadamia nuts, dill seeds, quinoa seeds, pistachio nuts, and sunflower seeds.

- **Oils**: coconut oil, flaxseed oil, almond butter, and olive oil are awesome sources of alkaline.

Acidic Foods to Avoid as Much as Possible

In order to remain in good health, be deliberate about avoiding the following.

If you have been used to eating these types of foods regularly, the temptation may be high to continue eating them, but the truth is that you are heaping a load of work for your body every time you consume them. If you cannot completely avoid them, then you should drastically cut down their consumption. They are considered the top acid-forming foods.

- Refined grains
- Processed meats (cold cuts)
- Processed foods (bread, rice, and pasta including packaged grain products)
- Processed cereals (corn flakes and the like)
- Junk foods

- Dairy (eggs, cow milk, and cream cheese)
- Alcohol and caffeine

Other Habits that can Increase Your Acidity

Aside from eating foods that are highly acidic, certain habits can equally contribute to increased acidity in your body. These include:

- Chronic stress
- Sedentary lifestyle (very high physical inactivity)
- Excess exercise
- Overuse of antibiotics
- Preservatives and food coloring
- Excess drug use
- Low fiber consumption

- Shallow breathing
- Exposure to herbicides, pesticides, and other pollutants

Precautions About Avoiding Acid-forming Foods

Eggs and cow milk are acid-forming? How come? Well, there are several other foods that you may be surprised to find on the acidic food chart, but that doesn't necessarily mean you should stop eating them completely. As a matter of fact, some of them contain omega 3 fatty acids and other antioxidants that are very useful for your body. Remember that I earlier mentioned that we are aiming for balance and not total elimination of acids from your body.

A Quick Word About Alkaline Water

When natural water like spring water travels over rocks, it picks up minerals along its journey and increases its alkalinity. This is alkaline water occurring naturally. But we don't have to go to a waterfall or spring with gallons to fetch alkaline water, do we? Certainly not! Electrolysis is a chemical process that is used to produce most of the alkaline water that you can easily buy in many grocery stores without necessarily traveling to a spring in search of natural alkaline water. However, be advised that not all alkaline water is produced using electrolysis. Distillation, reverse-osmosis and a few other methods can be used in the production of alkaline water, and some of these methods do not actually add mineral content to the water, nor do they raise the pH of the water. Ideally, alkaline water has a pH between 8 and 11, which makes it more alkaline. Pure water has a pH of 7, which makes it neutral.

Here's my take on alkaline water: it is safe to drink alkaline water as long as you do not overdo it to the point that it affects your stomach pH. Stomach acidity is necessary for effectively breaking down foods we eat. If you trust the manufacturer of the alkaline water and if you can afford to constantly buy it, then it is a great way to keep the body hydrated in an alkaline way.

However, you can drink distilled water. Adding a little bit of lime, lemon or even baking soda to your drinking water can raise the pH level. But whatever you do, avoid drinking bottled water and tap water.

The bottom line is to drink water that is not acidic (like tap water). Neutral water is just as good as alkaline water. If you drink freshly squeezed vegetable juices, you should get adequate amounts of alkaline-forming foods in your body. Keep in mind that your body's pH is not too far from the neutral pH level of 7, which is the pH of pure water. Drinking too much alkaline water may not be too ideal for your stomach health.

Perhaps now would be a good time to discuss the issue of excess alkalinity in the body.

Excess Alkalinity is Possible, But...

Okay, I know this is supposed to be a book that shows you how wonderful the alkaline diet is and all the amazing things you can benefit from by alkalizing your meals. Nevertheless, I'd be doing you a disservice if I do not point out the possible downsides of excess alkalinity. Remember that one of my goals in writing this book is to present you with a balanced perspective on the alkaline diet.

But is it possible to have excess alkaline in your body, especially with the rampant acidic foods enticing and urging us to consume them all the time? Well, yes. It is indeed possible to become overly alkalized. However, it is not for the reason you think! Excess alkalinity is not a common phenomenon in a world laden with so much sugar. Plus, it is a somewhat difficult thing for many people to significantly reduce their acidity let alone increasing their alkalinity to the extent of going overboard. Nevertheless, excess alkalinity is possible, and it is a health condition known as alkalosis.

There are different types of alkalosis which include metabolic, respiratory, hypokalemic, and hypochloremic alkalosis.

Metabolic alkalosis: a severe decline in body acidity or a significant increase in body alkalinity caused by diseases like kidney disease, adrenal conditions, excessive and prolonged vomiting can lead to metabolic alkalosis. Abusing diuretics (drugs that stimulate excess urine or that are used to rid the body of excess water) is also a factor that can eventually lead to alkalosis.

Respiratory alkalosis: this occurs when enough carbon dioxide in the body cannot be removed. Usually, this results from medical conditions that lead to hyperventilation like asthma, pneumonia, sleep apnea, and COPD. When one suffers from any lung or liver disease, it may also contribute to hyperventilation.

Hypokalemic alkalosis: when there is an acute shortage of potassium in the body it can lead to hypokalemic alkalosis. This is usually caused by diarrhea, excessive sweating, and some kidney conditions.

Hypochloremic alkalosis: when there is a drastic shortage of chloride in the body, perhaps due to severe vomiting over a long period of time, or a medical condition which causes profuse perspiration for a long time, it can result in hypochloremic alkalosis.

... It Has Nothing to do with An Alkaline Diet

Here's the thing: you cannot eat your way into excess alkalinity! In other words, following an alkaline diet would not make you have alkalosis, unless of course you just want to deliberately consume very insane amounts of highly alkaline foods consistently on a daily basis for a very prolonged period of time – something that is nearly impossible!

Go through the various causes of alkalosis again and see if there is any mention of consuming too many alkaline foods. Alkalosis is simply a medical term that describes a condition of excess alkalinity in the body, but that doesn't automatically translate to mean that it is caused by eating an alkaline diet or living the alkaline way.

So, go ahead and enjoy your alkaline foods; in fact, do not just end at "eating" alkaline alone but strive to "live" alkaline. A complete change in lifestyle should be your goal. That means you need to overhaul your eating habits (away with canned, sugary, and processed foods) as well other habits like excess workouts and stress-inducing activities. Do not be afraid to go green and help your body maintain its pH. Remember, excess alkalinity is possible, but it is not caused by eating an alkaline diet.

In Summary...

I'm sure you can now see that the alkaline diet goes far beyond weight loss. Maintaining the acid-alkaline balance of the body has numerous benefits, as we have seen in this chapter. Here is a brief recap.

- Reduction of inflammation, improving digestion, promoting healthy skin, and preventing respiratory problems are some of the health benefits of the alkaline diet.
- Consuming fresh vegetables as well as fruits, preparing and drinking fresh green juices, and eating plant-based proteins are good sources of alkaline-forming foods.
- As much as possible, steer clear of processed foods, junk foods (fast

foods), alcohol, caffeine, and processed meat.

• Some acid-forming foods have redeeming value and are vital for proper body functioning. Foods like eggs and milk, though acid-forming, can be taken moderately.

• Avoid habits like excessive workouts, antibiotic overuse, being physically inactive, and keep away from too much exposure to pesticides, herbicides, and other pollutants. They can cause your body to become highly acidic.

• Alkaline water is safe. Tap water is a no-no. Adding lime, lemon, or baking soda to your drinking water can raise its pH.

- Excess alkalinity is possible, but it is not caused by eating alkaline-forming foods.

Chapter 4: Medicinal Herb

Living a healthy life is a deliberate choice; it doesn't happen by accident, especially in this age and time when toxins can easily pass for food. Eating food is a way to replenish worn-out body cells and reinvigorate the body. Unfortunately, eating food is now one of the major ways to push the body into extreme conditions where diseases thrive. Thankfully, we can reinvent healthy eating by deliberately choosing what goes into our mouths. Alkalizing our meals is one way to accomplish this. Eating fresh vegetables or herbs will not just fill our stomachs, but serve as medicines to our bodies and keep us in a general state of good health.

It is difficult to discuss alkaline foods without mentioning herbs, since they play a very central role in maintaining good health. In this chapter, we shall take a look at what medicinal herbs are and how they can help to stimulate your body's natural healing process. Remember that we have earlier established in previous chapters that your body will do all it can to maintain its normal pH level, even if it means dumping acidic ash or waste into other organs. It does this to keep a regular blood pH level. By eating medicinal herbs, you help the body recover from toxicity and help to keep the internal environment unsuitable for germs to thrive. In other words, medicinal herbs are essentially preventive medicines; an effective way to keep diseases at bay.

What is a Medicinal Herb?

First of all, what do we refer to as herbs? Herbs are those plants that are used in part or whole as ingredients for adding flavor or fragrance to dishes. Medicinal herbs, on the other hand, are plants that are used for medicinal purposes. Medical herbs can be used for skin care, anti-inflammation, prevention of anxiety, anti-bacterial, soothing stomach upset, and so much more.

Herbs, unlike drugs, are not formulated. They are natural; freely given to us by mother earth and nurtured by water, air, and sun. The ancients relied on herbs for the treatment of ailments, nourishing the body, healing wounds, preventing diseases, and much more. But as time passed, we lost the knowledge of herbal medicine and turned to synthetic drugs and over-the-counter medicines for every ailment. We have forgotten that for every prescription medicine or treatment, there is a plant or herb (or some other natural substance) that can be effectively used instead of that prescription. And, as a matter of fact, herbalists and naturalists have been using these herbs for hundreds of years.

Medicinal Herbs versus OTC Medicine

Medicinal herbs are complete or whole foods containing curative effects. They are highly nutritious and filled with several minerals and vitamins that your body needs. This is why they treat a lot of symptoms at the same time. Medicinal herbs are also preventative, and they dig deep to the root cause of the imbalance in your body. You may take a medicinal herb to treat just one ailment but end up treating several other ailments because of the presence of vitamins and minerals.

OTC (over-the-counter) medicines, on the other hand, are band-aids that simply treat the effect and not the cause. They are good for quick, temporary relief, but usually have unpleasant side-effects. While it is true that many OTC medicines are sourced from plants, they often become tainted during all the processes they undergo in the lab before the final drug or medicine is available to the end-user.

Health Benefits of Medicinal Herbs

It takes a certain level of expertise to determine the combination of herbs that you will need for your health situation. Some herbs, or combinations of herbs, help with fever, skin problems, parasite removal, immunity, overheating, fatigue, liver function, and more. Here are a few benefits you can get from using medicinal herbs:

Anti-bacterial benefit: some medicinal herbs are known for having anti-bacterial capabilities. Fresh garlic, eucalyptus, clove, and thyme are some of the medicinal herbs that can prevent bacteria from growing in the human body.

Anti-inflammatory benefit: inflammation of the joints, nerves, stomach, muscles, and intestines can be effectively tackled with some herbs like cayenne, licorice, turmeric, and boswellia. These medicinal herbs basically decrease the activity of body cells that are pro-inflammatory in order to relieve irritation, pain, and stiffness.

Antispasmodic benefit: medicinal herbs like kava, cramp bark, valerian, and peppermint are great for treating muscle spasms without any adverse health effect on the sufferer.

Hepato-protective benefit: the liver is one vital organ in the human body that needs to be protected from damage that can arise from excess toxins in the body. Medicinal herbs like artichoke, dandelion, turmeric, and milk thistle serve to protect cells in the liver from damage. They equally support and promote normal liver function.

Carminative benefit: gas formation in the alimentary canal can be very discomforting. Fortunately, there are herbs that can prevent or, at the very least, reduce the formation of gas. These carminative properties can be found in herbs like ginger, fennel, peppermint, and chamomile.

Herbs and the Body's Natural Healing Process

In the same way foods support your body from a very basic level, herbs can do so too by stimulating your body's natural healing ability. You do not necessarily need to be an herbalist before you can use medicinal herbs. I have outlined some herbs and how they stimulate the natural healing process of the body. You can learn how to use them instead of developing an overdependence on synthetic drugs. Keep in mind that this is not professional medical advice. I strongly recommend that you consult with your doctor before applying any treatment, whether natural or synthetic.

1. **Ginger – prevents nausea**: ginger is known for its ability to ease nausea. Chemotherapy patients, as well as those suffering from motion sickness, have experienced significant improvements by using ginger. It is best to take ginger before experiencing nausea. As an example, if you get airsick whenever you travel by air, chewing gum

before your flight takes off can prevent nausea. However, if nausea has already set in, there are candies and even teas that contain ginger which can ease nausea.

2. **Lavender – helps to relieve stress and tension**: lavender oil is renowned for its relaxing and calming effect. Lotions and oils that contain lavender have aromatic properties that calm spasms, suppress pains, and alleviate insomnia, depression, anxiety, restlessness, and stress. Lavender oil is also used for:

- Relieving rheumatism and joint pains, tense or sore muscles, sprains, and backache. Massaging lavender oil on the affected area can bring about great relief.

- Improving digestion by stimulating the production of gastric juices and bile.

- Treating skin problems like eczema, acne, wrinkles, and psoriasis. Itchy skin and insect bites can also be soothed with lavender. It can help to keep moths and mosquitoes away, which is why some mosquito repellents have lavender oil as one of the ingredients.

- Maintaining healthy hair by boosting hair growth and also preventing nits, lice, and lice eggs.

1. **Chamomile – helps to promote sleep**: chamomile encourages sleep. Simply drink this herb as a warm tea to help you fall asleep and enjoy quality sleep.

2. **Ginseng – beefs up energy level**: this root is known to effectively fight off fatigue and in turn boost or stimulate your energy levels.

3. **Thyme – boosts production of antioxidants**: aside from providing nice fragrance to your dishes, thyme is known to contain a high level of antioxidants that help to bring relief from gastrointestinal and respiratory problems. It can also provide protection from toxins

that cause cancer. Thyme can also be used for:

- Improving oral health by using thyme oil as herbal rinses and mouthwashes.
- Preventing acne outbreaks as well as toning aged skin.
- Stimulating the mind, calming the nerves, and also strengthening memory.

1. **Fennel seed – relieves indigestion and bloating**: constipation and bloating can be treated using fennel seeds. You can ground the seeds and use them in teas.

2. **Licorice – soothes a sore**

throat: this root has anti-inflammatory properties that are capable of soothing a sore throat. Using it in teas will greatly relieve a sore throat.

3. **Cinnamon – controls blood sugar level**: adding cinnamon to your beverages and foods will go a long way toward keeping your blood sugar level in check. This is especially useful for people who have type II diabetes.

4. **Nettle – treats dandruff**: using this oddly named herb to wash your hair or as an addition to your shampoo can effectively treat dandruff. Drinking nettle leaves as tea or juice can help the body to

balance its acid-alkaline ratio. Fresh nettle is high in vitamin K, which makes it very effective in stopping most bleeding. Dried nettle, however, loses its vitamin K concentration.

5. **Mint – soothes upset stomach**: one medicinal herb that is considered very powerful in curing stomach aches is mint. To use this, simply drink it as a tea. It is also good as a diuretic and can be used for relaxation, too.

6. **Marigold – fights off wound infections**: marigold (also known as calendula) contains anti-inflammatory and anti-viral properties, which makes it an

excellent wound healing agent.

7. **Eucalyptus – eases lung congestion**: this plant is both a cleaning agent as well as an herb for treating lung problems. It clears mucus in the lungs due to its anti-inflammatory component. Keep eucalyptus essential oil by your bedside to help clear any congestion in your lungs.

8. **Parsley – combats bad breath**: due to parsley's high concentration of chlorophyll and vitamins, it is an excellent herb for treating bad breath. Eating it by itself, blending it in drinks, or using it to cook your meals are good ways to use parsley for fighting bad

breath.

9. **Garlic – boosts your immune system**: garlic has anti-fungal, antiviral, anti-bacterial, and immune-boosting effects. This makes it one of the richest medicinal herbs to have handy. Eating one or two cloves of fresh garlic on a daily basis may actually keep a whole lot of diseases away from you.

In Summary...

This book is about helping your body to reduce acidity and toxins; it is, therefore, important that we consider the natural ways which we can heal the body without adding extra chemicals that can cause unpleasant side-effects to our body. That is why this chapter covered some important lessons which included the following:

- Medicinal herbs help to stimulate the body's natural healing process.
- Herbs are natural and usually treat more than one disease or ailment due to their high vitamin contents.
- Synthetic drugs may provide temporary relief, but do not address the root cause of health problems.
- Herbs have natural anti-inflammatory, anti-bacterial, as well as antispasmodic health benefits, among others.

Chapter 5: Harvesting and Preparing Herbs

Harvesting

One of the ways you can escape the artificialness in most processed foods is by growing your own. I am not suggesting that you quit your job and become a farmer; however, owning a garden where you can harvest fresh herbs for your cooking needs is a great way to improve both your health and eating experience. You can equally grow specialty herbs that are relatively scarce at local markets and preserve them so that you can use them all year round.

Growing herbs is one thing; harvesting

herbs is a different ballgame entirely. All the efforts in planting and nurturing your delicate herb garden could go to waste if you do not know how and when to harvest the herbs and most importantly, how to preserve them. Getting the most out of herbs will mean harvesting them when they are at their peak freshness, and then storing them in the right way.

Although this is not compulsory to living the alkaline way, it is a good thing to equip yourself with the knowledge of harvesting and preserving herbs that will help you increase your likelihood of eating alkaline-forming foods. Growing your own herbs is one of the ways to encourage yourself (and those around you) to eat more vegetables, seeds, nuts, and even roots that are highly medicinal.

Best Times for Harvesting Herbs

The time to harvest any herb depends largely on what part of the plant is to be harvested (leaves, roots, seeds, or flowers) and what you intend to use the herb for. As a general rule, always harvest your herbs when there is ample foliage for maintaining the growth of the plant. If you have annual herbs on your garden, you can prune about 50 to 70% of the herb and they will recover just fine. For perennial herbs, removing one-third of the herb's growth at once is okay. For most culinary herbs, continuous pruning encourages new growth. When you cut or prune herbs, make sure to make clean cuts using a pruner or a sharp knife.

Leaves: ensure you harvest leaves of herbs like mint, basil, chives, parsley, and oregano before they flower. Pick them when they are still tender, because that is when they contain adequate amounts of oil that produce the best taste as well as fragrance. Harvesting leaves after they bloom or flower will make most herbs have an off-flavor. To stimulate continuous production of fresh new leaves, remove flowers as soon as they appear.

Roots: herb roots like chicory, goldenseal, ginseng, and bloodroot can be done after the foliage has faded. This would be towards the end of summer or around early fall.

Seeds: when harvesting herbs that are grown for seeds like fennel, cumin, coriander, dill, and caraway, ensure you harvest them as the seed pods begin to change to gray or brown.

Flowers: to harvest flowers like tarragon, chamomile, lavender, and borage, collect them right before they fully blossom.

On a general note, the best time of the day to harvest most herbs is in the morning when the dew has evaporated and before the day becomes hot. When you pick leaves, remember not to wash them unless you intend to cook them immediately. If you are not using them immediately, simply rinse them to remove soil and shake off the excess water before storing them. Washing leaves when you pick them will make them lose the aromatic oils in them.

Also, be sure that pesticides have not been sprayed on the leaves you are harvesting. There are a lot of insecticides and pesticides that are not safe to be used on herbs meant for eating. So, if you have a garden, ensure that you control plant diseases and insects using healthy and approved methods.

Methods of Preserving Herbs

So, you've harvested a bunch of herbs from your backyard garden. Congratulations! But you now have a new challenge: how are you going to preserve all the herbs since you most definitely cannot eat all of them at once? There are a few ways you can preserve your herbs so that you can use them anytime the need arises. However, keep in mind that to get the best taste from herbs, use them immediately after you harvest them. After harvest, most herbs tend to lose their aroma and flavor very quickly. Making use of herbs immediately after they are harvested would mean going to the garden every now and then to harvest your herbs, and that could be a cumbersome process.

You can preserve them for short-term (a few days to about 2 weeks) or long-term (up to a year or 2). Note that preserving herbs beyond 1 year may make them lose too much fragrance and taste. Ideally, you should use them within a year.

Short-term Preservation Methods

To avoid going to your garden every single time you want to make use of a herb, you can harvest them and preserve them for up to a week or two using the following methods:

For herbs that have long stems like parsley, cilantro, and basil, you can fill a glass with water and store them inside just like you would keep flowers that you cut. Simply trim them at their ends and place them inside a glass of water, and then place them on top of your counter in the kitchen. You can keep them fresh that way for about one week.

For other fresh herbs like thyme, chives, and rosemary, you can simply wrap them up using a damp paper towel before placing them inside an open plastic bag. You can equally use a perforated plastic bag, too. Store the bag containing the herbs inside the vegetable bin of your refrigerator. Remember not to rinse or wash the herbs until you are ready to use them. They can remain fresh and retain their original taste and flavor for up to a week or 2 when stored this way, but keeping them longer than that using this method may cause a loss in flavor.

To preserve herbs for a longer period, consider using long-term preservation methods like drying and freezing.

Drying Method

The most common method of preserving herbs is by drying. Basically, with leafy herbs that have long stems, you can simply tie them in bunches and them hang them out to air dry. But first, you'll have to rinse off any soil from the leaves, pick out damaged leaves, shake off excess water, and then hang them upside down in a dry, warm and ventilated area like a barn, garage, shed, or a well-ventilated attic. Use a paper bag to cover seed heads so that you can collect them when they fall. This also applies to low moisture, sturdy herbs like thyme, sage, rosemary, dill, parsley, and savory. It usually takes about 2 to 4 week for the herbs to become properly dried. Pluck off the leaves and store them (without chopping) in a container and tightly close the lid. You can grind or crush them right before you use them.

For herbs that have large, tender leaves and contain high moisture such as lemon balm, bay leaf, mint, basil, tarragon, and lemon verbena, quickly dry them after harvesting so as to prevent mold from developing. Pluck out the leaves from the stems and then dry them in a single layer on a window screen or any frame that is covered with netting. After 2 to 3 days, turn the leaves to ensure all sides are properly dried. When the herbs are properly dried (usually within a week), put them inside a container and close tightly until needed.

Drying herb seeds requires that you cut the stems of the herbs with their seed heads as soon as the color of the heads starts to turn brown. Hang the stems upside down covered with paper bags to collect the seeds as I have described earlier. Once dry, shake the seed heads to collect the seeds. Clean the seeds by laying them on a flat clean surface and then blowing air across them to remove chaff and debris. Make sure the seeds are completely dry before storing them in sealed containers to avoid developing mold.

Drying leaves in the sun will affect foliage color and is not recommended. I do not recommend oven or dehydrator drying. However, if you can control the temperature of these appliances, then you can use them. Ideal drying is by air drying or the use of very low heat. Keep in mind that when herbs are dried, the flavor is concentrated, so when using them for recipes that require fresh herbs, remember to use about ¼ of the amount required.

Quickly, let us consider the various

ways you can dry your harvested herbs.

Tray drying: this is most suitable for individual leaves or herbs that have short stems. Any frame with mesh will serve the purpose. Lay the herbs in one layer on the tray and place it in a well-ventilated, warm area. Make sure that the tray is not placed in the sun. You will have to turn the leaves occasionally to ensure that the leaves are dried evenly.

Dehydrator drying: to use a food dehydrator for drying herbs, check the appliance manual for settings and instructions. Make sure to keep the temperature very low.

Oven drying: to use an oven for drying herbs, you will have to monitor the temperature very closely. Keeping the oven temperature somewhere between 80 to 100° F and allowing the oven door to remain slightly open will make for an ideal drying temperature. Make sure you often check the drying progress and turn the herbs when necessary. Using the oven method may take as long as 4 hours before the herbs are completely dry.

Microwave oven: you can use a microwave oven to quickly dry herbs in small quantities. I strongly recommend that you take all safety precautions when using this method. Read and understand the recommendations of the appliance manufacturer before using the appliance for drying herbs. Thoroughly rinse the herbs and dab them with a kitchen towel to remove excess moisture before microwaving. If the herbs have excess moisture, microwaving them will result in cooking instead of drying. Do not place the herbs directly into the microwave; place them in between two paper towels before microwaving on high for between 1 to 3 minutes. Turn the herbs every now and then so that they will dry evenly. Keep the herbs on a rack after taking them out of the microwave to allow them to cool before storing them in a sealed container.

Freezing Method

Freezing herbs is a good way to preserve them. When you freeze herbs for preservation, their appearance may change, but that does not affect the flavor of the herbs. Also, note that frozen herbs are not quite suitable for garnishing; they are best suited for cooking.

Herbs like borage, dill, basil, chives, mint, sage, oregano, lemongrass, tarragon, thyme, and savory all freeze well and usually maintain their quality even up to 6 months when frozen. Before you freeze lemongrass and chives, remember to chop them, as they are thin and can freeze up quickly.

Here are a few ways you can use the freezing method to preserve your herbs:

Cube them: thoroughly rinse the

herbs and then chop them coarsely. Fill ice cube trays with water and place the chopped herbs into the trays. Place the ice cube trays inside a refrigerator to freeze. Once frozen, take the cubes from the tray and place inside a plastic bag and store inside the freezer. Take out individual cubes when you need to use them.

Blanch them: you can preserve fresh leafy herbs by blanching them in boiling water for a few seconds (between 30 to 60 seconds). Remove from the boiling water and then dip them in very cold water to quickly cool them. When cool, chop and place the leaves inside a sealed plastic bag and put inside a freezer.

Freeze them: this is pretty straightforward. Properly rinse the herbs and lay them in a single layer inside a pan after patting them dry with a kitchen towel or paper towel. Place the pan into a freezer. Once frozen, remove the herbs from the pan and place them inside a tight plastic bag or container. Store them inside the freezer until you are ready to use them.

Freeze in oil: one of the best methods to freeze herbs which I personally recommend is this one. The reason I say it is the best is this: fresh herbs can have their active enzymes dramatically altered when damaged or heated. Herbs frozen in cubes take longer to melt and incorporate during cooking than those frozen in oil. What this means is that when you put frozen cubed herbs into your sauce or whatever food you are cooking, the core of the ice cube takes a longer time to melt, while the outer herbs are already melted and overcooking. This makes them lose flavor. Here's how to freeze your herbs in oil:

1. Thoroughly rinse the herbs and chop them roughly.

2. Fill ice trays with the chopped herbs and top with olive oil or any natural oil. If the herbs are in large quantity, put them inside a food processor and add the oil to it before processing.

3. Place the ice cube tray in a

freezer.

4. Once frozen, remove from the ice cube tray and place the cubes inside a zipper-lock bag until needed.

An alternative (and better) way to use this method would be to skip the ice cube trays and place the oiled chopped herbs directly inside a zipper-lock bag and leave about an inch or so of open space while sealing the bag. Squeeze out any air inside the bag by flattening the bag before completely sealing the bag. Place the flattened bag of oiled herbs on a baking sheet or large plate and put inside the freezer. This will make it freeze faster and also melt faster because of the surface area to volume ratio.

Salt-Cure Method

One other method you can use to preserve your harvested herbs is by using salt. This is rather an old-fashioned method, but it has the advantage of producing salts that are herb-flavored, which means you can use the salt to season your dishes to give them the flavor of the herb.

To use this method, simply place the herbs between layers of salt. Kosher salt or sea salt can serve this purpose. Do not use iodized salt. Pour the salt into a container (for example, a plastic tub or a glass jar) to form the base layer. Put the herbs on the layer of salt and then pour more salt to cover the herbs. Now cover the container very tightly with a lid and keep it in your kitchen. You do not need to keep this in the fridge, as salt is used to preserve herbs in places where there is no refrigeration.

There is a more "modern" way to preserve fresh leafy herbs with salt! And yes, you will store them in a refrigerator. Here's how to do that:

1. Properly rinse your leafy herbs like basil, cilantro, oregano, sage, chives, parsley, or a combination of different herbs, and dry them with a kitchen towel.

2. Use a sharp knife to roughly chop the herbs. You can use a food

processor if you have large amounts of herbs to chop. But be mindful not to over-process the herbs when using a food processor, or else you'll end up with a soggy mass of herbs or even a paste!

3. Use the ratio 4:1 for adding the herbs and salt. That is to say, 4 parts herbs to 1 part salt. For example, you will need 1 teaspoon of salt to mix with 4 tablespoons of chopped basil. Note: Using 1 tablespoon of salt for 4 tablespoons of herbs will make the herb rather too salty. Use a teaspoon for measuring the salt.

4. Combine the herbs and kosher or sea salt inside a clean container.

Gently stir the mixture and cover the container tightly.

5. Store inside a refrigerator. This can stay fresh for up to a few months.

Note: this method makes the herbs salty. So, when it comes time to use the herbs for cooking, ensure that you first add the herbs to the food then taste it for saltiness before adding additional salt to your dish.

In Summary...

Here is a quick summary of what we've discussed in this chapter.

- Planting your own garden of herbs will encourage you to eat fresh foods.

- Harvest herbs early in the day before the weather gets hot

- Wash herbs only when you intend to use them immediately so that they'll not lose their aromatic oils.

- Do not use pesticides on your herbs.

- Properly preserving herbs that you have harvested will keep them fresh even after a long time.

- Drying, freezing, and salt-curing are good ways to preserve your herbs.

- Do not dry harvested herbs in the sun.

Chapter 6: Alkaline Diet and Weight Loss

We live in a world where acids abound even in the air we breathe, and to make matters worse, we continually consume foods and drinks that form acids in our bodies. This can lead to excess body weight. Weight gain is simply one of the ways which your body has devised to accommodate the excess acidity it is being constantly fed.

I am aware that many people will read this book mainly because they want to lose weight, so let me begin by first correcting some misconceptions about weight loss. Starting with the right mindset and ideas will help your weight loss journey.

- **"*I want to lose weight*" is another way of saying "*I want to be healthier.*"** This is why I have put a lot of emphasis on balancing the acid-alkaline levels of your body, because once that is taken care of, you will enjoy overall health and that should take care of weight loss, too. You essentially cannot separate weight loss from healthy eating and living. In other words, there is no shortcut to it; you cannot desire to lose weight and then apply the alkaline diet as if it were some magic pill or drug that will automatically shed off your unwanted weight after which you will return to eating acid-forming foods. You have to make a commitment to eating healthily if you truly want to have a permanent weight loss result.

- **Starvation and following stringent diet plans do not guarantee weight loss.** As a matter of fact, starving your body of food in the hope of losing weight can make your body system activate the starvation mode. In simple terms, when you deprive yourself of food for a long time (such as fasting for prolonged periods of time in the guise of losing weight), your body senses that there is a severe shortage in food supply, therefore, it automatically starts to cut down the amount of fat it burns in order to conserve energy. So, instead of burning fat, your body protects fat, thereby mitigating or significantly slowing down the rate at which you lose weight. I do not mean to discourage you from fasting; on the contrary, I encourage people to practice some form of intermittent fasting if they can. The point here is that you do not have to starve yourself before you lose weight.

• **Excessive exercise in and of itself will not make you lose weight.** You have to understand that there is a huge difference between building/maintaining muscles and burning of excess body fat. It is true that your body burns fat when you exercise, but without complementing exercises with adequate diet plans, you are simply putting round pegs in square holes! It is like someone who wants to exercise their way out of a bad eating habit and eat their way into building or maintaining muscles; it simply doesn't work. If losing weight is your goal, focus first on improving your diet (in this case, alkalizing your diet), and then complement it with regular exercise. If building or maintaining muscle is your goal, concentrate first on exercising, and then complement it with a good diet plan.

- **Effective weight loss does not come about by depriving yourself of delicious foods.** Feeling deprived only creates a longing or a strong urge for the food that is "off limits." Delete the word "deprive" from your mentality and in its place, use the word "substitute." So you are substituting unhealthy foods with healthy ones to help you in your quest for weight loss. Truth be told, for every unhealthy food you are used to eating, there is a perfect substitute that is very healthy!

- **Weight loss does not mean eating foods you do not enjoy.**

Get rid of the idea that you have to succumb to some unpalatable dishes in order to lose weight. It is true that you may not be comfortable at first with some of the alkaline-forming foods you are switching to, but that is normal since your taste buds have been used to something completely different. But that does not mean every healthy food tastes bad. It's just like the unhealthy foods you are used to eating; you do not agree with all of them. Some taste great, while others don't. The exact same thing applies to eating healthy alkaline-based foods; some will taste great to you while others won't. But do not box yourself in; be flexible. In fact, following an alkaline diet gives you room to be creative and flexible with your meals.

- **You are going to falter a few times.** It is normal to make mistakes here and there while you are in the business of working on your weight. What is not normal is to think that you will go through a diet program to lose weight without making a few mistakes. It is because of this wrong notion that many people beat themselves up when they don't make a beeline towards their goal. Simply dust yourself off and have another go at it when you falter and fall.

- **The process doesn't have to**

be complex to be effective. It is true that losing weight may not be as easy as it is presented on the pages of a book, but the process doesn't have to be very complicated or complex before it is effective. One of the things you will find with the alkaline diet and the prescribed process for losing weight is its simplicity. The simpler the process, the easier it is to understand and follow.

A Few Considerations Before You Begin

Do not skip this section in a bid to hurriedly get to the next section about how to lose weight. There are very important considerations you need to make before jumping into the exact steps required to shed weight using the alkaline diet. It is lack of patience to fully understand all that is required that makes people jump from one diet program to the other looking for quick fixes, shortcuts, and fad diets. The result is always a rebound, and they gain back whatever few pounds they manage to shed off. Therefore, I strongly suggest that you patiently read through the following before you begin.

A 50/50 Diet Does Not Work

It never has and it never will, so forget about consoling yourself in the false hope that eating healthily 50% of the time and then eating unhealthy foods for the remaining 50% of the time will have some positive effects. You are simply canceling out any effort or progress you have made. Stop making excuses and arguing for your limitations! Lack of time, money, or will-power may be easy excuses to throw around, but the fact remains that if you do not have a proper plan for your weight loss diet program, you are most likely not to make any significant progress. Having a concrete plan in place before you begin will make losing weight easy, fun, convenient, and affordable; after all, eating shouldn't be a difficult thing, right?

Watch Out for the "What-The-Hell" Effect

I have earlier mentioned that you will make mistakes and falter. Here's the thing about mistakes in diet programs: because of the rigid and strict rules about what to eat, when to eat, how to eat, and in what measure to eat, a lot of people find it very tasking to accomplish. Violating any of the rules tends to bring on a feeling of guilt that is very likely to push them down the path of complete derailment from the diet program. When a person believes that they have violated the rules of a diet, there is the tendency to simply continue with the violation, or at least they tend to repeat the violation. This is because they feel that since they have already broken the rules, there is no need to continue with it. This line of thinking is known as the "what-the-hell" effect.

However, the truth of the matter is that a few mistakes do not cancel every single bit of progress you have made. Humans do make mistakes; that's part of what makes us human to begin with. So do not allow the negative psychological effect of guilt derail you from following the alkaline diet for weight loss, even when you make mistakes or when you cheat. Guilt can push you into overeating, effectively countering your weight loss goal.

State Your Vision Clearly

Where are you now in terms of your eating habits? Where do you want to go from here? These are questions you need to answer in order to develop a concrete plan of action towards achieving your weight loss goals. If you do not know precisely where you are now in your eating habits, it is going to be very difficult to move forward in the direction of your goals because you may not know what direction is forward, since you do not know exactly where you are! Here's something you can begin to do for the next week to help you get clear about where you are and where you want to go from there:

Get yourself a journal (any book will do) and begin to write down what you eat and when you eat it. This will open your eyes to your eating habits or current diet style. It will help you to answer the important questions that clarify your vision. What did I eat today? Did I have breakfast or did I skip it believing it will help me lose weight? Am I eating well or starving myself? Do I settle down to eat or am I always eating on the run? Do I skip meals in the day time and heap my plate full at night? What is the content of my meals? Are they healthy foods or junk and processed foods?

Take the time to write down these and many more for just one week, and you will be able to clearly see your eating habits. This will give you a clear idea on what to improve, what to throw out completely, and what to include in your diet. You may even decide to continue with the journal beyond one week to help you keep track of your progress.

Create a Concrete Plan

Do not just wake up in the morning and rush to your meal plan to see what's on the menu for the day. That's not proper planning; in fact, that's a sure way to miss your target! Take out time every evening or night for at least 5 to 10 minutes to consider what you will require to prepare a healthy alkaline meal throughout the next day. Factor in your schedule for the next day (are you going to be very busy at work, in school, or are you going to be traveling?). Don't leave your preparations to chance – you are not going to figure it out as you go, because that attitude will lead to grabbing a few bites of fast food here and there. Ensure you understand what you will require for breakfast, lunch, and dinner. Make room for healthy alkaline snacks and take them along with you to avoid junk fast foods. Remember, you do not have to be a great cook or a master chef before you prepare healthy dishes. The alkaline diet gives you the option of making smart eating choices that can suit whatever your budget is.

How to Lose Weight using the

Alkaline Diet

Without further ado, here is exactly what you need to do to lose weight using the alkaline diet.

1. **Significantly decrease your sugar intake**. You'll have to bid farewell to refined sugars. Foods like low-fat yogurt, ketchup, sports drinks, protein bars, cereal bars, commercial produced smoothies (bottled smoothies), and canned fruits among others have high sugar content. Fruit, too, contain sugar, but you need the vitamins and minerals in them. However, keep fruit consumption very moderate.

2. **Increase your consumption**

of green plant foods. Eat a lot of spinach, watercress, chard, kale, wheatgrass, cucumbers, and parsley.

3. **Eat your greens mostly raw**. Eating raw vegetables, grinding them into a powdery form, or making them into smoothies are options you can explore and discover which works best for you. In their raw state, greens have a high negative charge, which makes them more alkaline – a quality that helps the free flow of energy throughout your body.

4. **Drink adequate amounts of**

water. Consider drinking alkaline water or making your own alkaline water by adding pH drops or lime to your drinking water. Even if you only take pure water, ensure that you are properly hydrated.

5. **Incorporate regular exercise**. You do not necessarily have to work out like someone preparing for the Olympics, but you do have to exercise a few times per week. 20 to 30 minutes of moderate exercise is good to get your heart pumping. If you can break a sweat, that's awesome, too. Remember that increasing your rate of respiration will go a long way in eliminating unwanted acids. Ensure

that you keep yourself hydrated after exercising. Hitting the gym is good, but if you can't do that for some reason, here are some ways you can become more physically active:

- Take a bus or public transport instead of riding in your car.
- Stop a few blocks from your destination and walk the rest of the way.
- Take the stairs instead of the elevator or lift.
- During weekends, take a walk in nature or around your neighborhood.

These are the steps you need to stick to consistently. Every other thing you will ever do to lose weight using the alkaline diet is summed up in the steps above. They appear simple, right? Well, do not be deceived by their simplicity. You will observe that the bulk of your work centers around what you eat, and that is because the plant foods listed above have an overabundance of qualities that help in normalizing your body weight.

Some of these qualities include:

- **Having high fiber contents**: this is essential to weight loss because fiber helps to discard unwanted matter from your body.

Please note that apples and bran are also sources of fiber, but since they can be acidifying, I do not recommend them for the purpose of weight loss.

- **Having a high level of magnesium**: magnesium is also necessary to make your heart pump properly to aid the elimination of unwanted matter.

- **Containing substantial amounts of chlorophyll**: these are the basic building blocks from which healthy red blood cells are formed. To effectively lose weight, your body needs to form healthy red blood cells.

- **Alkaline water makes you**

pee more: that's a very good thing, because it flushes acids out of your system.

Possible Objections

- **I don't like eating greens**. I get it, not everyone would like to consume green vegetables in large quantity, but how badly do you want to drop off those extra pounds?

- **Vegetables are hard to come by and preserving them is difficult**. You can easily get vegetables in abundance at a grocery store. You can even plant a garden where you plant, harvest, and dry your own vegetables. Alternatively, place an order for green power (in chapters 4 and 5, we looked at how to preserve herbs since they form a vital part of the alkaline diet. Kindly go back to these chapters if you skipped them).

- **I can't eat the required quantity of greens**. If you are afraid you won't be able to eat enough greens, don't worry so much. There's a simple way to go around that. Make them into delicious tasting smoothies! Before long, you'll be consuming large quantities of greens.
- **I really can't find the energy to exercise**. That's quite normal for

someone who is overweight. Excess acidity depletes your energy, so you won't feel the energy for physical activities. It is like a vicious cycle; you lack energy so you can't exercise, and the more you don't exercise, the more you lack energy! But here's the thing, once you begin to incorporate the alkaline diet by eating nutrient dense plants and drinking alkaline fluids, your energy levels will begin to rise. Before long, you will find that you are bubbling with a zest for life and you will eventually feel like moving your body around.

If You are not Getting Results...

In the unlikely event that results are not showing even after doing everything right, you need to consider the following factors:

- Are you on medication? Do you take oral contraceptives on a regular basis? Did you fit in a hormone-releasing coil? It is possible that some of your medications or contraceptives are messing with your system. If this is the case, you need to talk with a qualified physician with the aim of reducing your dosage or even completely putting a halt to it if that is possible. Drugs do have an acidifying effect on your overall pH level. Please do not alter your medications or contraceptives without proper medical advice from a qualified physician.

• Are you experiencing any emotional trauma? The habit of overeating can result from trying to hide from negative feelings about whatever situation is bothering you. If that is the case, you need to work on restoring your emotional health before embarking on any weight loss program.

• Do you hate your job? Do you feel purposeless? Are you just "drifting" in life? If you do not feel you have a purpose in your life or you appear generally lost about what it is you truly want from life, it can have negative impacts on your overall health. We may not readily accept the concept of spirituality, but there is no denying the fact of mind over matter. You may be unintentionally sabotaging your weight loss goals by the negative thoughts you hold in your mind. Consider taking some lessons in cognitive behavioral therapy (CBT) to help in correcting your internal negative chatter.

But wait! Is this process of losing weight not missing something? Shouldn't you be counting calories? Can you lose weight effectively without counting calories? Isn't it necessary to reduce your caloric intake when trying to lose weight? Let's briefly consider this before bringing this chapter to a close.

Should You Count Calories?

First of all, understand that the term "calorie" as it applies to diet simply means the measure of the energy value of foods. Every food has a calorie measurement; some small and others large.

It is often taught that you need to count your calories if you want to lose weight. That is to say, calculate your energy needs (using an online calculator or some other means) and then decrease the number of calories by 500 or more to reduce your weight. Also, you'll have to be very mindful of your food portion, get a kitchen scale (probably a digital kitchen scale for precise measurement) to measure your food, look at the label of every single food item to determine its calorie count before consuming, take every single snack into consideration - in short, if it is going into your mouth, you have to write it down!

Are you surprised that many people simply give up on many weight loss programs? It is a very cumbersome process to begin to keep track, record, and scale everything we eat. Eating food is supposed to be a fun process – a process you enjoy and not a process that makes it feel as if you are performing a job you don't like.

It is okay to balance your nutrients; eating only one type of food, for example, only foods that are rich in protein, may not be healthy for you over the long run. The right meal is one that takes balance into consideration. It is called a balanced diet because the basic nutrients (carbs, fat, and protein) are in the right proportions. I have discussed this earlier in chapter 2 under the heading, **Alkalizing Your Diet: The Process**. Please flip back there if you haven't already read it.

Losing weight has been put forward as *burning more calories than you eat*. So, most people who are into a diet program tend to focus on eating fewer calories. But that is absolutely the wrong way to focus. Instead of concentrating on calories, turn your attention to what you consume - simple!

Basically, there are two types of foods we consume:

Type 1: Those foods that the body can make use of; extracting nutrients from them and using them to replenish itself and ensuring that you thrive as a living human being. These are foods like low-sugar fruits, vegetables, fresh foods, healthy fats and oils, seeds, nuts, leaves, and salads. These are basically alkaline foods that are antioxidant-rich, anti-inflammatory, have a high water content, and are generally nutrient-dense.

Type 2: Those foods that the body needs to cope with; reacting to them, processing them, and trying to recover from them. These are foods like refined foods, sugar, trans-fats, junk foods, fast foods, pastries, sweeteners, sweets, chips, bread, and grains. In other words, these foods are acidic, capable of spiking up your blood-sugar level, oxidizing, inflammatory, and hormone-depleting.

Eat foods in **Type 1** and you will be in a generally healthy state and lose weight fast! But if you ignore that and eat foods in **Type 2**, your body will be under intense pressure to cope and deal with these food types. While you will not collapse and die from eating highly acidic foods (at least not immediately), if you continue eating highly acidic foods for a long time, your body will continue to do its best to keep you alive but you will also have to cope with symptoms like weight gain, loss of libido, skin conditions, arthritis, fatigue, etc. These are side effects of putting your body under undue pressure for a long time.

A Quick Challenge

Here's a challenge I'd like you to try. For the next 7 days, include just one alkaline meal in your diet. And to make that easy for you, I have listed below 7 delicious alkaline recipes that are super simple to prepare. In the next chapter, I have included a 7-Day Meal Plan that contains complete alkaline meal plans you can use for breakfast, lunch, and dinner for 7 consecutive days. Use that to kick-off your alkaline diet (for weight loss and general health) but for now, test the waters with this simple once-in-a-day alkaline meal.

First Day: Overnight Oats

Prepare this the night before. Simply pour a ½ cup of oats in a jar. Add 1 tablespoon of ground flaxseed, chopped dates or bananas, and sprinkle some pumpkin seeds on top. Pour in 1 cup of coconut, almond, or oat milk. Cover the jar and keep it in the fridge. The milk is absorbed overnight. Overnight oats can last up to 3 days in the fridge, so you can increase the size by 3 and store it in the fridge to provide you with 3 days of delicious breakfasts.

In the morning, simply take out your overnight oats, grab a spoon, and eat your delicious breakfast. Add more water (alkaline water preferably) or more milk if the oats are too dry. For extra creaminess and taste, you can add fresh berries.

Second Day: Cauliflower Roast

Take a whole cauliflower and cut it into large florets. Put the cuts into a baking tray and toss in some chopped garlic, sliced onions, green beans, and some diced chicken (for protein). Drizzle the ingredients with some olive oil and season with pepper and salt to taste. Roast for about 45 minutes over medium-high heat. Stir occasionally so that the vegetables cook evenly. You can eat this as lunch or dinner.

Third Day: Green Smoothie

Mix the following into your blender:

½ cup coconut milk or almond milk; 1 cup of spinach (firmly packed); 1 teaspoon of spirulina powder; 1 small peeled and pitted avocado; freshly squeezed juice of half a lemon; 2 ice cubes, and a pinch of salt.

Blend together until the mixture is smooth. You can add a little bit of water if the smoothie is too thick.

Fourth Day: Stuffed Date Snack

Find some good, big, succulent, and dark dates. Take out the stones from inside your dates and stuff them with whole almonds. Store them in a Tupperware box and use as a snack.

Fifth Day: Avocado Salad (Nutty and Lemony Variation)

Pour 2 cups of kale inside a saucepan with 1 inch of hot water. Allow steaming with the lid on for about 5 minutes over low heat. While that is boiling, gently heat ½ tablespoon of oil and add some seeds and nuts like pumpkin seeds and walnuts. Take out the nuts when they begin to turn brown and place them inside a paper towel to remove excess oil.

Grate 1 carrot into a bowl and add ½ courgette to it. Add sliced avocado, cooked kale, and the nuts into the bowl. Squeeze some fresh lemon juice into the bowl and drizzle with avocado oil. Season with pepper and salt to taste and enjoy! You can eat this alone or with brown rice.

Sixth Day: Sweet Potato Soup

Peel and dice 3 sweet potatoes. Boil them in a pan over medium heat until soft. While that is cooking, slice and fry half an onion with 3 cloves of garlic over medium heat until soft.

Now put the sweet potatoes and some of the boiled water into a blender. Add in the fried onion and garlic, plus a little raw ginger. Also, add ground cardamom (½ teaspoon), and ground cinnamon (½ teaspoon). Now blend the mixture until smooth on a low-medium speed.

Pour the blended mixture back into the pan and allow it to simmer for about 10 minutes over low heat. You can season it with salt and pepper and also add some coconut milk if you want.

Seventh Day: Spelt Pasta with Pesto

Follow the instructions on the spelt pasta packet to cook it. While that is cooking, prepare your homemade pesto by adding a handful of basil and pine nuts into a blender. Add in 1 clove of garlic and sprinkle some vegan parmesan on it. Blend the ingredients while slowly adding olive oil, and then season with salt and pepper when a creamy consistency is reached.

Mix the pasta with the pesto and enjoy with some steamed broccoli. You can increase the measure for the pesto and store in a fridge for five days.

Keep in Mind...

You may experience some form of inconvenience and become uncomfortable, especially at the initial stages of beginning your weight loss journey using the alkaline diet. This is absolutely normal. Your body is adjusting itself to expel more acidity from tissues and organs, so a bit of pain may be experienced. It is possible to also experience digestive upsets. These are not signs or symptoms that the alkaline diet is not good for you. Simply continue to consume alkaline-forming foods, focusing more on green vegetables and lowering your sugar intake as much as possible. This is why it is a good idea to ease into this diet, especially if you have been neck-deep in consuming highly acidic food your entire life. I strongly encourage you to start with the 7-day challenge and gradually increase your alkaline intake until you can completely change your diet.

Discomforts are expected, and they should fade away in a short while. However, if the symptoms persist beyond the first and second weeks, I strongly recommend that you consult a qualified dietician or a physician who is experienced in issues relating to body pH balance. Also, if you do have any underlying health challenge or you are currently under any medication, it is best to consult your doctor and discuss the possible suitability of switching your diet at this point in your life.

In Summary...

This chapter is probably the main attraction for a lot of people reading this book. The weight loss process presented here may appear ineffective at first glance because of its apparent simplicity. However, rest assured that it works! And to drive home the main points, here is a recap of what we have covered in this chapter.

- Do away with the misconception that weight loss diets must be complex, difficult, and strenuous in order to be effective. The simpler the process, the easier it is to understand and apply.

- At the root of weight loss is the need to stay healthy. Focus on eating healthily, and you will be well on your way to achieving the weight of your choice.

- Mistakes will happen along the way; it is a normal occurrence. Dust yourself off and continue eating healthily.

- Do not give up on your goal because you violated a rule. Feeling guilty can lead you to overeating and return you right back to where you began.

- Spell out your vision in clear terms. Use a diet journal to help you define exactly where you are and where you want to be. This will help you create a concrete action plan.

- To lose weight, decrease your sugar intake and increase your green vegetable consumption, especially in raw form. Remain hydrated by drinking alkaline water or adding lime to your water, and engage yourself in some regular physical activity.

- If it seems like results are not forthcoming, check to see that you are not sabotaging your efforts through medications, negative emotional habits, and a general lack of life purpose.

- Discomforts may occur especially at the beginning of your weight loss diet program. It is normal. However, do consult a doctor if the symptoms persist.

- Counting calories is not necessary to lose weight. It is a cumbersome process that I do not recommend as it is likely to make you "*throw the baby out with the bathwater!*"

- Do the 7-day challenge!

Chapter 7: The 7-Day Alkaline Meal Plan

Important Note

Please note that some of these recipes (especially breakfast recipes) require prior preparation of ingredients the night before. Therefore, take your time to study the recipes a day or two beforehand so that you will make adequate preparation plans.

Day 1

Breakfast: Chia and Strawberry Quinoa

Lunch: Sweet and Savory Salad

Dinner: 3 ounces of roasted Chicken

with Roasted Sweet Potatoes and Parsnips

Breakfast: Recipe and Preparation (Chia and Strawberry Quinoa)

Ingredients

- 5 tablespoon chia seeds
- 1 cup cooked quinoa
- 4 sliced strawberries
- 2 tablespoon almonds (chopped)
- 2 pitted dates
- 1 ½ cup coconut milk
- ½ cup quartered strawberries
- coconut flakes (unsweetened, shredded)

Directions

1. Cook the quinoa. Use a blender to prepare a puree of dates and coconut milk. All this should be done the previous night.

2. Into a jar, pour the mixture and add the chia seeds, then thoroughly mix.

3. Place a lid over the jar and allow it to refrigerate overnight.

4. By morning, put the chia seeds and quinoa inside a bowl and add toppings. Breakfast is ready!

Snack: If you feel like snacking before lunchtime, eat an orange.

Lunch: Recipe and Preparation (Sweet and Savory Salad)

Ingredients

- 1 avocado (cubed)
- 1 head of butter lettuce (washed)
- 1 pomegranate (seeded)
- ½ cucumber (sliced)
- ¼ cup shelled pistachios (chopped)

Dressing Ingredients

- 1 garlic clove (minced)
- ½ cup extra virgin olive oil
- ¼ cup apple cider vinegar

Directions

1. Cut the butter lettuce and place in a bowl.

2. Add in all the other ingredients. Garnish with dressing and serve.

Snack: for the snack option, dried fruits alongside a half cup of toasted nuts will do.

Dinner: Recipe and Preparation (Sweet Potatoes and Parsnips)

Ingredients

- 1 ¼ pound sweet potatoes (chopped into small pieces of about ½ inch thick)
- 1 ¼ pound parsnips
- 1 tablespoon Dijon mustard
- 2 tablespoons olive oil
- 2 tablespoons maple syrup
- parsley (chopped)
- ground pepper and coarse salt

Directions

1. Set your oven to 450° F and allow to preheat
2. Peel the parsnips and cut

3. Place the parsnips on a large baking sheet (rimmed). Toss in the chopped sweet potatoes. Add olive oil, pepper, and salt.

4. Spread well to cover just one layer and allow it to roast for about 30 minutes. Wait until golden and tender. Remove and place inside a large bowl.

5. Mix the mustard and maple syrup together in a small bowl. Pour the mixture on the vegetables and let it coat.

6. Sprinkle some parsley over it and serve.

Day 2

Breakfast: Vegan Apple Parfait

Lunch: Savory Avocado Wraps and White Bean Stew

Dinner: 3 ounces of roasted Chicken and roasted Brussels sprouts with Red Peppers

Breakfast: Recipe and Preparation (Vegan Apple Parfait)

Ingredients

- ½ cup raw cashews (soaked for between 20 minutes to 1 hour)
- ½ teaspoon vanilla extract
- ½ cup unsweetened coconut milk
- 1/3 cup uncooked rolled oats
- 1 tablespoon hemp seeds
- 1 cup apple (chopped)

Directions

1. In a blender, put in vanilla, coconut milk, and cashews. Blend until a smooth consistency is achieved.

2. Pour the cashew cream in a cup to form the bottom layer, then put the chopped apples as the next layer, followed by the hemp seeds and oats as the top layer.

3. Serve and enjoy your healthy breakfast!

Snack: Feel like snacking? Eat one pear before lunch.

Lunch: Recipe and Preparation (Savory Avocado Wraps and White Bean Stew)

For the Savory Avocado Wraps

Ingredients

- 1 collard leaf bunch or butter lettuce
- ½ avocado
- ¼ red diced onion
- 1 teaspoon basil (chopped)
- 1 teaspoon chopped cilantro
- 1 sliced tomato
- spinach (small handful)
- pepper and sea salt

Directions

1. Place the avocado on top of the

collard leaf or lettuce and then add toppings of spinach, sliced tomato, cilantro, and the other ingredients. Season with salt and pepper.

2. Fold the leaf in half and enjoy the wraps.

For the White Bean Stew

Ingredients

- 2 garlic cloves (chopped)
- 2 cans cannellini beans (rinsed and drained)
- ¼ cup extra virgin olive oil and another ½ tablespoon extra virgin olive oil
- 1 ¾ cups chicken broth
- 5-ounce baby arugula
- 8 slices baguette

- 14 ounces of tomatoes
- ¼ teaspoon black pepper

Directions

1. In a pot, cook the chopped garlic with ¼ cup of extra virgin oil for between 1 to 2 minutes over medium to high heat.

2. Cut the tomatoes roughly and toss into the oil.

3. Stir in the beans and broth with black pepper and allow the mixture to boil.

4. Reduce the heat and uncover the pot. Allow simmering for 5 minutes.

5. Add in the greens and allow it to cook for between 1 to 3 minutes

until wilted.

Snack: Instead of going for some fast food or processed snack, keep a handful of toasted pumpkin seeds handy for a snack before dinner is ready.

Dinner: Recipe and Preparation (Brussels sprouts with Red Peppers)

Ingredients

- 1 ½ pound small Brussels sprouts
- 4 tablespoons extra virgin olive oil
- 1 red bell pepper (diced in small pieces)
- 2 garlic cloves (minced)
- 1 tablespoon grated lemon zest
- 1 tablespoon chopped mint
- Salt

Directions

1. Cut the bottom edges of the Brussels sprouts. Take off and set

aside unattached leaves.

2. Cut the sprouts in half and put in a bowl. Add salt to taste and add 1 tablespoon of olive oil.

3. Use parchment to line a sheet pan. Set oven to 400° F and allow to heat.

4. In a large skillet placed over medium-high heat, heat 2 tablespoons of olive oil.

5. Add in Brussels sprout halves (as many as can fit one layer) ensuring that the cut side is faced down and allow it to sear for about 3 to 5 minutes when it becomes brown.

6. Remove from heat and place on a baking sheet with the cut side

down. Repeat the same process for the remaining Brussels sprouts. Now place the baking sheet in the oven to roast for about 10 minutes until the sprouts become tender.

7. In the meantime, pour the remaining oil in a pan and heat over medium heat. Add in red pepper and stir often while it cooks for 5 minutes until it becomes tender. Toss in the garlic and allow it to cook for another minute while stirring.

8. Put in the roasted Brussels sprouts and mix thoroughly. Mix in the mint, lemon zest, and pepper. Add seasoning to taste.

9. Remove from heat. Allow it to

cool a bit before serving.

Day 3

Breakfast: Berry Purple Smoothie

Lunch: Chicken Sesame Noodle Salad

Dinner: 4 ounces Roasted Salmon, ½ baked Sweet Potato, Curried Beets and Greens

Breakfast: Recipe and Preparation (Berry Purple Smoothie)

Ingredients

- 2 cups fresh spinach
- 2 cups homemade almond milk
- 1 tablespoon chia
- 1 peeled banana (frozen)
- 1   cup

mixed berries, strawberries (frozen)

- 4 tablespoon raw almond butter

Directions

1. First, put the spinach in a blender and add almond milk. Blend together.

2. Add other ingredients excluding chia and blend until smooth.

3. Now add chia into the blended mix and blend again, this time at low speed.

4. Allow the mixture to sit for a few minutes so that the chia seeds will expand.

5. Serve your smoothie and enjoy!

Snack: if you get really hungry before lunch, take one healthy mango as a snack.

Lunch: Recipe and Preparation (Chicken Sesame Noodle Salad)

Ingredients

For the dressing

- ¼ cup white vinegar (distilled)
- ¼ cup natural peanut butter
- 1/3 cup soy sauce
- ½ cup coconut oil
- 1 tablespoon minced ginger
- 2 tablespoons sesame oil
- 2 tablespoons water
- 2 cloves garlic (peeled)
- 2 tablespoons honey
- lime juice (a few squeezes)

For the salad

- 4 ounces brown rice noodles
- 1 pound chicken breast (boneless, skinless)
- ½ cup peanuts or cashews
- 1 cup cilantro leaves (packed, chopped)
- 5 cups spinach or baby kale
- 3 large carrots (cut in small pieces)
- 3 bell peppers (cut in small pieces)
- 4 green onions (chopped, green parts only)

Directions

1. Put rice noodles in a bowl containing cold water and allow it to soak.

2. Set oven to preheat at 400° F.

3. Except for the peanut butter, pulse every other ingredient for dressing in a food processor.

4. Put the skinless boneless chicken breast in a plastic bag and marinate it with the peanut butter. Place inside a refrigerator for between 15 to 30 minutes.

5. To the dressing inside the food processor, add some peanut and pulse. Set aside.

6. Prepare all the vegetables and mix in a bowl.

7. Take the marinated chicken out of the fridge and bake in the oven for about 15 to 20 minutes. Take out of the oven and allow it to cool

down for about 5 minutes then slice and put inside the bowl of vegetable mixture.

8. Remove the soaked noodles from water and drain before placing in a skillet. Allow it to cook over medium to high heat.

9. Add some oil and a little dressing. Mix and allow softening. If necessary, add some water.

10.   Toss the noodles along with the vegetable mixture and baked chicken. Garnish it with cilantro and crushed cashews or peanuts. Serve and enjoy.

Snack: go for a handful of dried apricot if you feel like snacking before dinner.

Dinner: Recipe and Preparation (Curried Beets and Greens)

Ingredients

- 1 bunch beet greens
- 1 tablespoon coconut oil
- ¼ cup finely chopped stems
- ½ finely chopped onion
- ½ serrano chili
- ½ teaspoon ground cumin
- ½ teaspoon turmeric
- ¼ semolina
- ½ teaspoon chili powder
- 1 tablespoon lemon juice
- 1 cup water
- 3 cloves garlic
- salt (to taste)

Directions

1. Set stove to medium heat. Pour oil in a skillet and heat.

2. Toss in garlic, chopped onions, beet stems, and chili.

3. Allow cooking until onions become transparent.

4. Add in the semolina and stir for about 3 minutes until it starts to smell toasty.

5. Add cumin, turmeric, and chili powder and stir.

6. Now pour in a little water, beet greens, and some salt.

7. Cover and allow it to cook for about 5 minutes. Stir a few times.

8. Remove the cover and cook for another 5 minutes while stirring.

9. Remove from heat and drizzle

some lemon juice over it. Stir and
serve.

Day 4

Breakfast: Apple and Almond Butter Oats

Lunch: Green Goddess Bowl

Dinner: Kale Pesto Zucchini Noodles

Breakfast: Recipe and Preparation (Apple and Almond Butter Oats)

Ingredients

- 2 cups oats
- 1/3 cup raw almond butter
- 1 cup green apple (grated)
- 1 ½ cups coconut milk
- cinnamon powder

Directions

1. The night before, place the coconut milk with oats and almond butter in a bowl and mix thoroughly.

2. Add the grated apple and stir. Place inside a jar that has a lid and put inside a fridge overnight.

3. By morning, remove from fridge and sprinkle a dash of cinnamon powder on it. Serve and enjoy!

Snack: eat one banana for a snack.

Lunch: Recipe and Preparation (Green Goddess Bowl)

Ingredients

For avocado cumin dressing

- 1 avocado
- 2 freshly squeezed limes

- 1 cup water (filtered)
- 1 tablespoon cumin powder
- 1 tablespoon extra virgin olive oil
- ¼ teaspoon sea salt
- dash cayenne pepper
- ¼ teaspoon paprika (smoked, optional)

For tahini lemon dressing

- ¼ cup tahini
- 1 tablespoon extra virgin olive oil
- ½ cup water (filtered)
- ½ freshly squeezed lemon
- 1 clove garlic (minced)
- black pepper
- ¾ teaspoon sea salt

For salad

- 3 cups chopped kale
- ½ spiralized zucchini
- ½ cup chopped broccoli florets
- 1/3 cup cherry tomatoes (halved)
- 2 tablespoon hemp seeds
- ½ cup kelp noodles (soaked and drained)

Directions

1. Steam the broccoli and kale lightly. Set aside.

2. Mix the kelp noodles together with the zucchini noodles. Add a good quantity of smoked avocado cumin dressing. Add in the halved cherry tomatoes and toss.

3. Place the broccoli and steamed kale on a plate and sprinkle some lemon tahini dressing. Use the tomatoes and noodles to top the greens.

4. Sprinkle with hemp seed. Serve and enjoy!

Snack: go for a handful of almonds. They make a perfect snack!

Dinner: Recipe and Preparation (Kale Pesto Zucchini Noodles)

Ingredients

- 1 bunch kale
- 2 cups fresh basil
- ¼ cup extra virgin olive oil
- ½ cup walnuts
- 2 freshly squeezed limes
- sea salt and pepper
- 1 spiralized zucchini (noodled)
- garnish with tomato, spinach leaves, and sliced asparagus (optional)

Directions

1. Soak the walnuts the previous night.

2. Add all the ingredients together in a blender and blend until a creamy consistency is achieved.

3. Add the mixture to the zucchini noodles. Serve and enjoy!

Day 5

Breakfast: Power Smoothie

Lunch: Quinoa Burrito Bowl

Dinner: Wild Rice Mushroom Risotto

Breakfast: Recipe and Preparation (Power Smoothie)

Ingredients

- 2 cups homemade almond milk
- 2 cups fresh spinach
- 2 tablespoons raw almond butter
- 1 banana (frozen)
- 1 cup mixed berries (frozen)
- 1 tablespoon coconut oil
- ½ teaspoon cinnamon

Directions

1. First, add the spinach and almond milk in a blender and blend.

2. Add the other ingredients and continue to blend until the mixture is smooth.

3. Serve and enjoy!

Snack: for the snack option, having an avocado between breakfast and lunch is a great idea!

Lunch: Recipe and Preparation (Quinoa Burrito Bowl)

Ingredients

- 2 15 ounce cans of adzuki bean (or black beans)
- 1 cup quinoa

- 1 heaped teaspoon cumin
- 2 freshly squeezed limes
- 2 sliced avocados
- 4 garlic cloves (minced)
- 4 green onions (sliced)
- chopped cilantro (a small handful)

Directions

1. Cook the quinoa according to the instructions on the package.

2. While the quinoa is cooking, warm the black beans in a large skillet over low heat.

3. Stir in cumin, garlic, onions, and lime juice. Allow cooking for about 10 to 15 minutes.

4. Divide the quinoa and use the

fresh cilantro and sliced avocado for topping. Serve and enjoy!

Snack: if you feel like snacking, reach for a handful dates.

Dinner: Recipe and Preparation (Wild Rice Mushroom Risotto)

Ingredients

- 1 tablespoon extra virgin olive oil
- 1 ½ cup wild rice (uncooked)
- 1 ½ cups celery (chopped)
- 2 garlic cloves (minced)
- 2 cups vegetable broth
- 4 white mushrooms (medium sized, sliced)
- ½ yellow onion (chopped)

- ½ cup green onions (sliced)
- ½ cup pecan halves (raw)
- salt and pepper

Directions

1. In a medium or large pan, sauté the onion, mushrooms, garlic, and 1 cup of celery. Stir often until celery and onion become tender.

2. Pour in the vegetable broth. Add the wild rice and allow the mixture to boil.

3. Reduce heat and allow it to simmer for about 1 hour while the pan is covered until the rice becomes tender. Stir very well halfway into cooking.

4. Remove from heat when rice is

cooked and uncover the lid.

5. Add the green onions and the remaining ½ cup of celery and mix.

6. Use a parchment paper to line a baking sheet. Set your oven to 350° F.

7. Spread the pecans and allow them to toast for about 8 minutes. Remember to flip halfway through.

8. Chop the toasted pecans and add them to the risotto.

9. Serve and enjoy!

Day 6

Breakfast: Chia Breakfast Pudding

Lunch: Miso Soup with Fermented Tofu

Dinner: Roasted Root Vegetables with

4 ounces of salmon

Breakfast: Recipe and Preparation (Chia Breakfast Pudding)

Ingredients

- 1 tablespoon coconut flakes (unsweetened, shredded)
- 1 cup coconut milk
- ½ teaspoon cinnamon
- ½ teaspoon vanilla extract
- 4 tablespoon chia seeds
- ¼ cup chopped nuts (hazelnuts, cashews, or almonds)

Directions

1. In a mason jar, mix chia seeds with milk the night before. Add the chopped nuts with cinnamon and

vanilla.

2. Cover the jar with a lid and shake thoroughly to combine the mixture. Place in a refrigerator overnight.

3. Take out of the refrigerator by morning. Shake very well and serve. If you choose, you can also add some more chopped nuts, coconut shreds, or fresh fruits.

Snack: for snack today, get a half cup of blueberries while waiting for lunch.

Lunch: Recipe and Preparation (Miso Soup with Fermented Tofu)

Ingredients

- ¼ cup firm fermented tofu

(cubed)

- ¼ cup nori (cut into somewhat large rectangles)
- ½ cup Swiss chard (chopped) or any other tough green
- ½ cup green onion (chopped)
- 4 cups water
- 3 tablespoon white miso paste

Directions

1. Pour the water into a medium saucepan and simmer.

2. Add the nori and allow it to cook for about 5 to 7 minutes.

3. Meanwhile, take a small bowl and add 3 tablespoons of miso with a small quantity of hot water. Whisk together. Now add it to the soup

and stir well.

4. Add all the other ingredients to the saucepan and allow them to cook for an additional 5 minutes.

5. Adjust seasoning to your taste. Remove from heat. Best served warm.

Snack: feel like eating something before dinner time? No worries. A handful of macadamia nuts will serve perfectly well.

Dinner: Recipe and Preparation (Roasted Root Vegetables)

Ingredients

- ½ cup olive oil
- 1 pound unpeeled red-skinned

potatoes (scrubbed and diced into small pieces)

- 1 pound peeled celery root (cut into small pieces)
- 1 pound peeled rutabagas (cut into small pieces)
- 1 pound peeled carrots (cut into small pieces)
- 1 pound peeled parsnips (cut into small pieces)
- 2 leeks (pale green and white parts only, sliced to 1-inch thickness)
- 2 tablespoons fresh rosemary (chopped)
- 10 peeled garlic cloves
- 2 onions (diced)

Directions

1. Place 1 rack in the center of your oven and another rack in the bottom third of the oven. Now set the oven to 400° F to preheat.

2. To prevent the vegetables from sticking, use olive oil to coat two baking sheets.

3. Except for the garlic, put all the other ingredients into a large bowl and combine. Toss to coat.

4. Use ample amounts of pepper and salt to season. Share the vegetables between the two sheets and roast in the oven for about 30 minutes while occasionally stirring.

5. Reverse the positions of the baking sheets. Add 5 peeled garlic cloves to each of the baking sheets

and to roast for another 45 minutes. Remove from oven when it turns golden and soft.

6. Serve and enjoy!

Day 7

Breakfast: Quinoa Porridge

Lunch: Mexican Quinoa Salad

Dinner: Pumpkin Soup

Breakfast: Recipe and Preparation (Quinoa Porridge)

Ingredients

- 1 can coconut milk (15 ounces)
- 1 teaspoon cinnamon
- ½ cup quinoa (rinsed)
- 1 teaspoon chia seeds
- 1 teaspoon hemp seeds

Directions

1. Except for the hemp seeds, add

all ingredients into a small saucepan and simmer for between 10 to 15 minutes when all liquid is absorbed.

2. Spread the hemp seeds on top and serve.

Snack: grab a few slices of cantaloupe if you feel the need to snack before lunch.

Lunch: Recipe and Preparation (Mexican Quinoa Salad)

Ingredients

- 1 can pinto beans (15 ounces), rinsed and drained
- 1 can kidney beans, (15 ounces) rinsed and drained
- 2 cups quinoa (cooked)

- 1 cup brown rice (cooked)
- 1 red onion (chopped)
- 1 red bell pepper (chopped)
- ¼ cup fresh cilantro (chopped)
- 1 can corn (14 ounces, optional)

Dressing

- 1/3 cup red wine vinegar
- ¾ cup olive oil
- 2 cloves garlic (mashed)
- 1 tablespoon chili powder
- ½ teaspoon salt
- ¼ teaspoon cayenne pepper
- ½ teaspoon ground black pepper

Directions

1. In a glass container with a lid, mix quinoa, cilantro, brown rice, red onion, red bell pepper, kidney beans, and pinto beans together.

2. Thoroughly mix the dressing and pour it over the quinoa mixture. Toss to coat.

3. Place the lid over the container and place the mixture in a refrigerator for about 2 hours so that the flavors will blend well.

4. Remove from refrigerator and enjoy!

Snack: I'll recommend a handful of dried coconut slices for a snack.

Dinner: Recipe and Preparation (Pumpkin Soup)

Ingredients

- 2 sugar pumpkins
- 2 shallots (diced)
- 3 cloves garlic (minced)
- 2 cups vegetable broth
- 1 cup light coconut milk
- 2 tablespoon honey or maple syrup
- ¼ cinnamon
- ¼ nutmeg
- ¼ teaspoon sea salt
- ¼ black pepper

Directions

1. Use parchment paper to line a

baking sheet as you set your oven to 350º F to preheat.

2. Cut off the tops of the sugar pumpkins with a sharp knife and cut them into halves. Scrape out the seeds and strings using a sharp spoon.

3. Use oil to brush the flesh and place them on the baking sheet faced down.

4. Allow them to bake for about 45 to 50 minutes until the skin can be easily pierced by a fork.

5. Remove from oven and allow them to cool for about 10 minutes. Peel off the skin and set aside.

6. In a large saucepan placed over medium heat, pour in 1 tablespoon

of olive oil, garlic, and shallot. Cook for up to 3 minutes.

7. Add all the other ingredients and the pumpkin, and then let it simmer.

8. Pour the soup into a blender and puree. Return the mixture back to the saucepan.

9. Cook for another 5 to 10 minutes over medium to low heat. You can adjust the seasoning as desired.

10.   Best served hot!

In Summary...

Here's the 7-Day Meal Prep at a glance - without the ingredients and directions, of course!

Day 1

Breakfast: Chia and Strawberry Quinoa

Lunch: Sweet and Savory Salad

Dinner: 3 ounces of roasted Chicken with Roasted Sweet Potatoes and Parsnips

Day 2

Breakfast: Vegan Apple Parfait

Lunch: Savory Avocado Wraps and White Bean Stew

Dinner: 3 ounces of roasted Chicken and roasted Brussels sprouts with Red Peppers

Day 3

Breakfast: Berry Purple Smoothie

Lunch: Chicken Sesame Noodle Salad

Dinner: 4 ounces Roasted Salmon, ½ baked Sweet Potato, Curried Beets and Greens

Day 4

Breakfast: Apple and Almond Butter Oats

Lunch: Green Goddess Bowl

Dinner: Kale Pesto Zucchini Noodles

Day 5

Breakfast: Power Smoothie

Lunch: Quinoa Burrito Bowl

Dinner: Wild Rice Mushroom Risotto

Day 6

Breakfast: Chia Breakfast Pudding

Lunch: Miso Soup with Fermented Tofu

Dinner: Roasted Root Vegetables with 4 ounces of salmon

Day 7

Breakfast: Quinoa Porridge

Lunch: Mexican Quinoa Salad

Dinner: Pumpkin Soup

Chapter 8: The Acid-Alkaline Food Chart

To give you different perspectives, I've included 3 acid-alkaline food charts in this chapter. These charts are designed by expert nutritionists: Dr. Russel Jaffe, Julie Cove, and Robert O. Young. If you are reading this on a device like your phone or computer, you may need to zoom in to see the chart text more clearly.

A first glance at the charts may make it appear complex to follow or understand, but do not worry too much about knowing every single food or drink on the chart all at once. You will get the hang of it as you refer to it regularly with time.

Chart 1 the pluses (+) and minuses (-) will guide you in choosing what to eat from chart 1. A plus sign means the food or drink is alkaline – more pluses on a column mean a higher alkaline level, and you should consider eating more of such foods. A minus sign means the food or drink is acidic – the more minuses on a column mean a higher acidity level, and you should keep away from such foods.

Chart 2 contains a list of foods that range from highly alkaline to highly acidic. It is very important to significantly cut down the foods listed on the moderately acidic list and do everything possible to avoid the highly acidic foods.

Chart 3 presents a more specific food acidity (-) or alkalinity (+) per ounce of food (this is an approximate value though). The higher the alkalinity (+) the more you would want to consume such food. The lower the alkalinity (meaning a higher acidity indicated by a - sign) the less you would want to consume such food. I have broken Chart 3 into 3 pages for convenience sake and to make it easy to read.

Refer to this chart from time to time, especially when you are preparing your food shopping list.

Chart 1

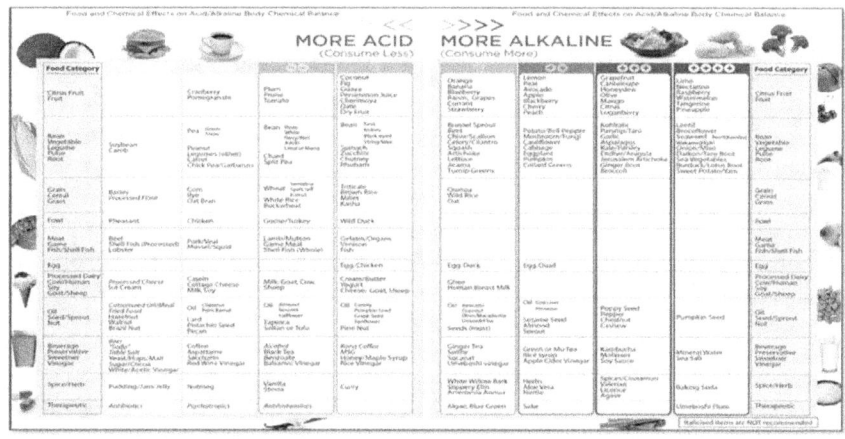

Image source: https://www.drrusselljaffe.com/wp-content/uploads/2016/11/dr.-russell-jaffe-alkaline-chart.png

Chart 2

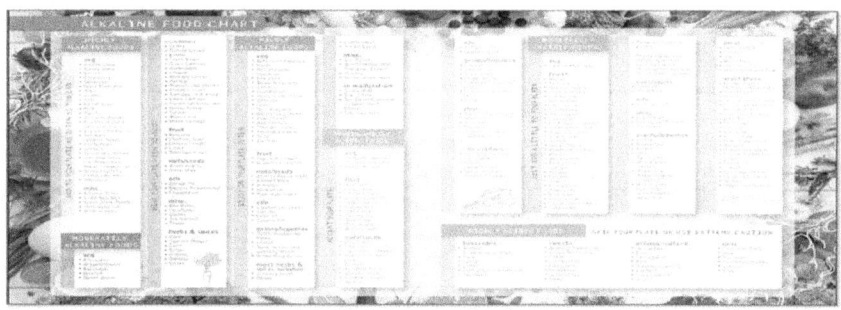

Image source: http://www.alkalinesisters.com/wp-content/uploads/2010/01/alkaline-food-chart-from-my-book.jpg

Chart 3

Alkaline Foods Chart

Healthy Alkaline Foods
Eat lots of them!

Foods you should only consume moderately

Unhealthy Acidic Foods
Try to avoid them!

Vegetables
Alfalfa Grass +29.3
Asparagus +1.3
Barley Grass +28.1
Brussels Sprouts +0.5
Cabbage Lettuce, Fresh +14.1
Cauliflower +3.1
Cayenne Pepper +18.8
Celery +13.3
Chives +8.3
Comfrey +1.5
Cucumber, Fresh +31.5
Dandelion +22.7
Dog Grass +22.6
Endive, Fresh +14.5
French Cut Green Beans +11.2
Garlic +13.2
Green Cabbage December Harvest +4.0
Green Cabbage, March Harvest +2.0
Kamut Grass +27.6
Lamb's Lettuce +4.8
Leeks (Bulbs) +7.2
Lettuce +2.2
Onion +3.0

Fruits
(In Season, For Cleansing
Only Or With Moderation)
Apricot -9.5
Bananna, Ripe -10.1
Bananna, Unripe +4.8
Black Currant -6.1
Blueberry -5.3
Cantaloupe -2.5
Cherry, Sour +3.5
Cherry, Sweet -3.6
Coconut, Fresh +0.5
Cranberry -7.0
Currant -8.2
Date -4.7
Fig Juice Powder -2.4
Gooseberry, Ripe -7.7
Grape, Ripe -7.6
Grapefruit -1.7
Italian Plum -4.9
Mandarin Orange -11.5
Mango -8.7
Orange -9.2
Papaya -9.4

Meat, Poultry, And Fish
Beef -34.5
Chicken (to -22) -18.0
Eggs (to -22)
Liver -3.0
Ocean Fish -20.0
Organ Meats -3.0
Oysters -5.0
Pork -38.0
Veal -35.0

Milk And Milk Products
Buttermilk +1.3
Cream -3.9
Hard Cheese -18.1
Homogenized Milk -1.0
Quark -17.3

Bread, Biscuits (Stored
Grains/Risen Dough)
Rye Bread -2.5
White Biscuit -6.5
White Bread -10.0
Whole-Grain Bread -4.5

content/uploads/2010/01/alkaline-food-chart-for-sit.gif

Peas, Fresh +5.1
Peas, Ripe +0.5
Red Cabbage +6.3
Rhubarb Stalks +6.3
Savoy Cabbage +4.5
Shave Grass +21.7
Sorrel +11.5
Soy Sprouts +29.5
Spinach (Other Than March) +13.1
Spinach, March Harvest +8.0
Sprouted Chia Seeds +28.5
Sprouted Radish Seeds +28.4
Straw Grass +21.4
Watercress +7.7
Wheat Grass +33.8
White Cabbage +3.3
Zucchini +5.7

Root Vegetables
Beet +11.3
Carrot +9.5
Horseradish +6.8
Kohlrabi +5.1
Potatoes +2.0
Red Radish +16.7
Rutabaga +3.1
Summer Black Radish +39.4
Turnip +8.0
White Radish (Spring) +3.1

Fruits
Avocado (Protein) +15.6
Fresh Lemon +9.9
Limes +8.2
Tomato +13.6

Peach -9.7
Pear -9.9
Pineapple -12.6
Rasberry -5.1
Red Currant -2.4
Rose Hips -15.5
Strawberry -5.4
Tangerine -8.5
Watermelon -1.0
Yellow Plum -4.9

Non-Stored Grains
Brown Rice -12.5
Wheat -10.1

Nuts
Hazelnuts -2.0
Macadamia Nuts -3.2
Walnuts -8.0

Fish
Fresh Water Fish -11.8

Fats
Coconut Milk -1.5
Sunflower Oil -6.7

Whole-Meal Bread -6.5

Nuts
Cashews -9.3
Peanuts -12.8
Pistachios -16.6

Fats
Butter -3.9
Corn Oil -6.5
Margarine -7.5

Sweets
Artificial Sweetners -26.5
Barley Malt Syrup -9.3
Beet Sugar -15.1
Brown Rice Syrup -8.7
Chocolate -24.6
Dr. Bronner's Barley
Dried Sugar Cane Juice -18.0
Fructose -9.5
Honey -7.6
Malt Sweetner -9.8
Milk Sugar -9.4
Molasses -14.6
Turbinado Sugar -9.5
White Sugar -17.6

Condiments
Ketchup -12.4
Mayonaise -12.5
Mustard -19.2
Soy Sauce -36.2
Vinegar -39.4

Image source: http://www.alkalinesisters.com/wp-content/uploads/2010/01/alkaline-food-chart-for-sit.gif

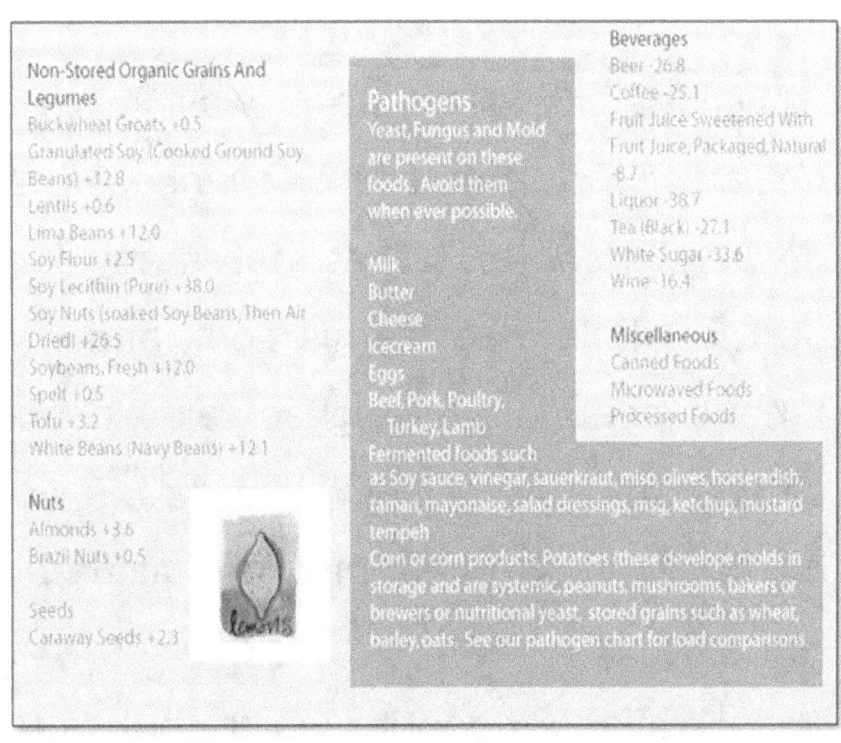

Non-Stored Organic Grains And Legumes
Buckwheat Groats +0.5
Granulated Soy (Cooked Ground Soy Beans) +12.8
Lentils +0.6
Lima Beans +12.0
Soy Flour +2.5
Soy Lecithin (Pure) +38.0
Soy Nuts (soaked Soy Beans, Then Air Dried) +26.5
Soybeans, Fresh +12.0
Spelt +0.5
Tofu +3.2
White Beans (Navy Beans) +12.1

Nuts
Almonds +3.6
Brazil Nuts +0.5

Seeds
Caraway Seeds +2.3

Pathogens
Yeast, Fungus and Mold are present on these foods. Avoid them when ever possible.

Milk
Butter
Cheese
Icecream
Eggs
Beef, Pork, Poultry, Turkey, Lamb
Fermented foods such as Soy sauce, vinegar, sauerkraut, miso, olives, horseradish, tamari, mayonaise, salad dressings, msg, ketchup, mustard tempeh
Corn or corn products, Potatoes (these develope molds in storage and are systemic, peanuts, mushrooms, bakers or brewers or nutritional yeast, stored grains such as wheat, barley, oats. See our pathogen chart for load comparisons.

Beverages
Beer -26.8
Coffee -25.1
Fruit Juice Sweetened With Fruit Juice, Packaged, Natural -8.7
Liquor -38.7
Tea (Black) -27.1
White Sugar -33.6
Wine -16.4

Miscellaneous
Canned Foods
Microwaved Foods
Processed Foods

Image source: http://www.alkalinesisters.com/wp-content/uploads/2010/01/alkaline-food-chart-for-sit.gif

Conclusion

My opening statement was *"Staying healthy is not a matter of chance - it is a deliberate choice."* That statement sums up the whole idea of this book and what I have been discussing so far. You can either put yourself in charge of your health by eating healthily, or succumb to the whims and caprices of an uncontrollable appetite which makes you susceptible to every kind of disease and illness.

It is entirely up to you to choose between good digestion and acidifying your system. We do need acids in our body to ensure balance; however, we live in a time and age where a high percentage of what we consume as foods and drinks are highly acidic, causing a shift in the balance that our bodies rightfully deserve. This lopsidedness makes our system overwork itself in a bid to restore its natural balanced state. The result? Too much strain on your body. This can only mean that illnesses are not far away from such a strained body system.

The alkaline diet may be fraught with misconceptions here and there, but no one can deny the efficacy of low-sugar fruits, vegetables, and herbs in general. I have carefully taken a non-sentimental middle path to present to you the very rudiments of how to take advantage of the alkaline diet to improve your overall health and well-being. This is why I have included a comprehensive section about herbs to show you the various ways you can use them as preventive measures against diseases.

Keep this book handy as a go-to guide. That means you'll probably have to read it over and over again, concentrating on sections you need to fully understand or apply. As you do so, do not forget to create a 5 minute daily routine (for at least 30 days) to test your pH level using either your saliva, urine, or both. This is one way that you will know how your body is performing.

You may have been attracted to the alkaline diet because you simply want to lose weight fast! That's a noble goal, but I'm sure by now you would have realized that losing weight is only one benefit of following the alkaline diet. While it is a good idea to reduce your alkaline food intake when you observe a balance in your body pH, I strongly recommend that you make eating an alkaline diet a lifestyle change. Following a diet to lose weight then returning to your old habit of eating is a huge waste of your own time and effort. You will most definitely gain back the weight. Say your goodbyes to your old ways of eating and embrace a new lifestyle, where you recognize that your best medicine is your food!

References

1. Allen, M. (2018). 8 Healing herbs for anxiety, inflammation, and more. https://www.byrdie.com/healing-herbs

2. Bridgeford, R. (2016). The simple weight loss equation (…if you're counting calories you have to read this). https://liveenergized.com/alkaline-diet-resources/the-simple-weight-loss-equation/

3. Bridgeford, R. (2018). Can you get too alkaline? https://liveenergized.com/alkaline-diet-resources/too-alkaline-alkalosis/

4. Bridgeford, R. (2019). Losing massive weight with the alkaline diet.

https://liveenergized.com/alkaline-diet-resources/weight-loss-alkaline-diet/

5. Cove, J. and Becker, Y. (2010). Alkaline foods chart. http://www.alkalinesisters.com/alkaline-food-chart/

6. Daily Health Post (2019). 7 Day alkaline diet plan to fight inflammation and disease. https://dailyhealthpost.com/alkaline-diet-plan/2/

7. DYLN Inspired (2018). Alkaline diet plan for weight loss. https://www.dyln.co/blogs/y-blog/alkaline-diet-plan-for-weight-loss

8. Elkaim, Y. (2019). The alkaline acid

food chart (use this to rejuvenate your health). https://yurielkaim.com/alkaline-acid-food-chart

9. Encyclopedia.com (2008). Berthelot, Pierre Eugène Marcellin https://www.encyclopedia.com/people/science-and-technology/chemistry-biographies/pierre-eugene-marcellin-berthelot

10. Felicetti, M. J. (2019). How to balance your pH to heal your body. https://www.mindbodygreen.com/0-6243/How-to-Balance-Your-pH-to-Heal-Your-Body.html

11. Frothingham, S. (2018). What is the pH of saliva? https://www.healthline.com/health/ph-

of-saliva#risks

12.   Gioffre, D. (2016). How to correctly test your ph levels. https://www.getoffyouracid.com/blogs/ph-info/how-to-correctly-test-your-ph-levels

13.   Hernandez, L. (2017). Salt preserved fresh herbs: Simple ingredients, endless possibilities. https://www.kitchenstewardship.com/salt-preserved-fresh-herbs/

14.   IG Smart Home Improvements (2017). Can your body have too much alkaline? https://www.intelgadgets.com/blog/can-your-body-have-too-much-alkaline/

15.	Jaffe, R. (2019). Dr. Russell Jaffe alkaline food chart. https://www.drrusselljaffe.com/alkaline-food-chart/

16.	Jaffe, R. (2019). 7 Principles of eating the alkaline way. https://www.drrusselljaffe.com/7-principles-eating-alkaline-way/

17.	Laleva.org (2004). Louis paste£ur vs Antoine Béchamp and the germ theory of disease causation – 1. http://www.laleva.org/eng/2004/05/louis_pasteur_vs_antoine_bchamp_and_the_germ_theory_of_disease_causation_1.html

18.	Leech, J. (2018). The alkaline diet: An evidence-based review.

https://www.healthline.com/nutrition/the-alkaline-diet-myth

19.   Levy, J. (2018). Alkaline diet: The key to longevity and fighting chronic disease?   https://draxe.com/alkaline-diet/

20.   Link, R. (2017). 15 Acidic foods to avoid + healthier alternatives. https://draxe.com/acidic-foods/

21.   Lopez-Alt, J. K. (2015). Freeze fresh herbs for long-term storage. https://www.seriouseats.com/2015/03/how-to-freeze-herbs-for-long-term-storage.html

22.   Mercola, J (2014). 7 Underrated medicinal   plants.

https://articles.mercola.com/sites/article
s/archive/2014/09/01/medicinal-
plants.aspx

23.   Pike, C. (2015). 4 Healing herbs
for   healthy   skin   &   body.
https://eminenceorganics.com/ca/blog/2
015/03/13/4-healing-herbs-healthy-
skin-body

24.   Scearce, J. (2019). 20 Amazing
uses for herbs to heal your body and
mind.
https://www.lifehack.org/articles/lifestyl
e/20-amazing-uses-for-herbs-heal-your-
body-and-mind.html

25.   Turner, N. (2017). How to
balance your pH and find out if you're
too   acidic.

https://www.chatelaine.com/health/diet/
tired-overweight-you-might-be-too-
acidic/

26. Turner, N. (2014). Four reasons to take a break from booze. https://www.chatelaine.com/health/deto x-health/health-reasons-to-stop-drinking-alcohol/

27. University of Illinois Extension (2019). Harvesting, drying and storing herbs.
http://extension.illinois.edu/herbs/tips.cf m